FACIAL

AND

HOMEOPATHY

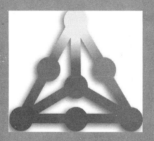

Fulfilling Hahnemann's Legacy

Grant Bentley

An imprint of
B. Jain Publishers (P) Ltd.
USA - EUROPE - INDIA

FACIAL ANALYSIS AND HOMEOPATHY

First Asian Edition: 2011
6th Impression: 2020

First published 2003/2006 in Australia by Grant Bentley

For Sale within Asia and Africa (Except Japan)

Published by Kuldeep Jain for
B. JAIN PUBLISHERS (P) LTD.
B. Jain House, D-157, Sector-63,
NOIDA-201307, U.P. (INDIA)
Tel.: +91-120-4933333 • *Email:* info@bjain.com
Website: **www.bjain.com**

Printed at: Nice Printing Press

ISBN: 978-81-319-1826-5

INTRODUCTION

Facial Analysis and Homeopathy is two books joined together and forms the underpinning development and knowledge that is known as Homeopathic Facial Analysis (HFA). The two books were published in the last decade

Appearance and Circumstance – 2003

Homeopathic Facial Analysis – 2006

Some upgrades and minor changes have been incorporated into this book but essentially it represents the majority of work from *Appearance and Circumstance* and *Homeopathic Facial Analysis*. My third book *Soul & Survival* – 2008 is a continuation of the HFA clinical work and details my interpretation of our defence mechanism (miasm) and how it is linked to inherited memory.

Facial Analysis and Homeopathy details the development of HFA from its humble beginnings as an attempt to both interpret but more importantly clinically use the concept of a miasm as a working diagnostic. HFA has surpassed my greatest imaginations as a clinical tool and is the foundation of not only my homeopathic practice but that of a growing number of HFA practitioners worldwide.

HFA has given me what I could only dream of as a new student and then practitioner and teacher – a measurable objective way of using the foundations of Hahnemann's miasm theory. Although I have developed and reworked his original disease theory I am indebted to the genius of this man who laid out every brick of the foundation to allow me to build the HFA system.

The cases for each miasmatic group are presented in their original form but the graph software has been upgraded to RadarOpus – the rubrics are the same as originally used.

The acknowledgements, dedications and introductions remain in their original form as written in both 2003 and 2006.

Grant Bentley – November 2011

A scorpion wanted to cross a river so he asked a frog if he would carry him.

"No," replied the frog, "for if I let you on my back you might sting me, and the sting of a scorpion means certain death."

"Now where," asked the scorpion, "is the logic in that? For if I were to sting you, I would drown."

Convinced, the frog allowed the scorpion on his back. But then, in the middle of the river, the frog suddenly felt a terrible pain and realised that the scorpion had stung him.

"Why did you sting me?" asked the frog. "For now we will both surely die?" "I know," replied the scorpion, "but frog, I am a scorpion. It's my nature."

Proverb

ACKNOWLEDGEMENTS
(Appearance and Circumstance 2003)

I would like to thank all my patients. Every Homoeopath understands that the clinic is the real teacher. No new information can be gained without experimentation and so with much appreciation I say thank you for your trust and acceptance.

To my students, many of whom have been with me as this project developed, for your endurance to put up with all the confusion and for allowing me to use you as a sounding board for ideas, – thanks to you all.

To everyone that was willing to help by allowing their photographs to be displayed, thank you so much.

I would also like to thank Kent Homeopathic Associates; the research for this book could never have been accomplished so quickly if it were not for their software. Also thanks to Greg White for his help and technical advice.

To Allan Cornwell thanks for your help in making this book become a reality.

To my mother Betty, for her understanding and help and to my father Keith who recently passed away. I would have loved you to see this.

To Jill and Noel for their help, interest and encouragement.

To my step children Katie, Sophie and Emma. Thanks for your help and understanding. Having to be quiet so often was difficult I know but it helped heaps. Thanks for your understanding and interest too.

To my children Lauren, Andrea, Sally and Jack a big thank

you for your love, support, enthusiasm and all your questions. I hope I can give to you as much as you have given me.

Finally to my partner Louise without whom this book would not exist. Your support has been boundless and your encouragement unending. You gave love, patience and understanding at times when a response of exhaustion or frustration would have been more appropriate. On a practical level you have contributed by always knowing the right questions to ask and your development of the triangle as a way to highlight the miasms has helped enormously. Your valuable contributions to the facial features such as the asymmetrical nature of blue to take just one example have become trustworthy guides. For taking on extra duties so I would be free to give the book my full attention, the list is endless! For these reasons and many more with all my love, respect and appreciation, I dedicate this book to you.

DEDICATION

For Louise

CONTENTS

Appearance and Circumstance 2003

INTRODUCTION
(Appearance and Circumstance 2003)

A book is the culmination of a thousand different ideas and theories. Often they begin with nothing more than a faint flicker, a "what if" or a throwaway line. Most of the time, very little comes from these postulations, but occasionally one idea won't go away it keeps building and evolving until it takes off like a wildfire and develops a life of its own; this book is the result of one of these ideas.

I would love to you tell a tale of development like that of Newton and the apple tree or Galileo and the pendulum, a precise moment of time when an idea was conceived. Perhaps a case of serendipity? A chance occurrence where one's perspective is changed forever. But such a story would be untrue, for the development of this miasmatic model had humble origins. The truth is, I am uncertain as to how it all started - but it did and now I find the way I practice Homoeopathy has changed, and the world has become a far more interesting, yet at the same time understandable place in which to live. The development of this miasmatic model has been the single greatest learning tool in my understanding of Homoeopathy and life in general. What started as an attempt at understanding a few more remedies has become a way of life, a guiding philosophy that helps me understand why things happen and to whom they are most likely to occur.

In the past I knew the Miasms were important only because Hahnemann had said so, however for much of the time they were seldom applied in practice. Miasms played little part in the process of case taking and even less in remedy selection. Patients with distinctly Syphilitic backgrounds were receiving doses of Nat Mur for their depression or perhaps Sulphur because they looked unkempt or were philosophical. Others were being administered Aurum because of a sense of responsibility even though their spirit was as light as helium. I look back in horror at many of my past prescriptions, cases that I can now see clearly then screaming out their miasm but falling on ears as deaf as a post. Today as my results show, I can tell a different story, one of vastly improved accuracy and professional confidence, a story where as a practitioner I am in control of the case from start to finish. I don't always get it right of course, but my chances have significantly improved and this is solely due to miasmatic awareness and categorisation method.

As a lecturer of Classical Homoeopathy, I am in a privileged position. Not only am I constantly reviewing Materia Medica, but I frequently re-read texts like the Organon, Kent's Lectures and other traditional works. I know well Hahnemann's story, his twelve years of labour formulating the doctrine of the Miasms. At its conclusion, Hahnemann believed he had the answer to what lies behind all chronic illness, a working model that, in his opinion explained the balancing act between health and illness. Here, thought Hahnemann, was the answer to that most allusive of medical questions; "why do we get sick?"

Things happen when they are meant to. Year after year I read the Organon in class with students when one day, the bell rang. To understand the miasms is to understand what sickness is, as miasms and disease are one and the same thing, there is only one true sickness in any individual's life and that is the miasm that dominates them. Everything else is simply how that miasm manifests; this starting point highlighted three major questions;

1. What is a miasm?

2. How do I recognise it?

3. What do I do with it?

The development of this model is based on my attempt to answer these three questions. These questions have consumed me for the last five years, an obsession that has reached at times almost maniacal proportions. There were times when I wished I could drop the whole idea, and still others where I would become so thoroughly confused I was convinced that the model was either fundamentally flawed or just plain wrong. Then something new would fall into place and a new piece of the puzzle would unfold to show that the information was accurate, but incomplete. Enthusiasm would rekindle, awe would follow and the whole process would start again. Its beginnings were modest, no thoughts of lectures, much less a book, the drive was an effort to be a better Homoeopath and to understand, as much as one individual can, this system that we all admire and love so much.

There are always fears and reservations when venturing into new ground, and even more about presenting new ideas publicly, but the remarkable increase in the precision of my constitutional prescriptions provides a confidence that allows me to do so. Nonetheless there are some uncertainties I would like to address. These include:

1. **Miasmatic themes.** There was some hesitation as to how much detail a miasmatic theme should contain. By design a Homoeopathic theme is an attempt to standardise individual characteristics for easier

recognition. But it sometimes can reduce temperament to a cliché profile. A theme is a premise, a foundation on which other facts are built. The problem with personality profiles as a foundation is they are not concrete, they are just one demonstration of an assortment of possibilities and as a consequence, themes can lead you astray if you view them as set rather than flexible. Themes may shift and yield, like the water in our remedies, and as a consequence take on and mould itself to an influencing character. For example, Arsenicum is a remedy of many varied keynotes; fastidiousness being only one of them, however to expect to see this trait in every Arsenicum case is just as naive as expecting fastidiousness to always be associated as neatness. This will lead to as many failures as successes. At the same time many wonderful cures have only been made possible by drug pictures such as "Mr. Arsenicum". In much the same way clinical cases have both exposed and confirmed distinct miasmatic issues. These issues often belong not solely, but certainly disproportionately, to a particular miasmatic group. These themes or issues are best understood if viewed as drives or energies rather than caricatures. This energy will influence decision making and can often be most accurately seen via events and patterns continually recurring throughout an individual's lifetime. Rather than portraits, miasmatic themes symbolize a power or quality that lies behind the conditions and actions that take place in accordance to the laws of attraction and repulsion. They are magnets that draw equivalent people, happenings and dramas.

2. **Varying opinions.** There are a number of ways miasms

can be interpreted many of which are different to what I am submitting in this book, but that is to be expected, after all, for a method to be new, it must differ from that which came before it. However no creation is ever entirely original and this book is no exception, it builds upon foundations laid down long before I took my first breath. I will show, by highlighting passages scattered throughout the Homoeopathic classics that many other authors were arriving at the same conclusions in reference to miasmatic understanding. One of the main principles in the book is the theory that there is a single dominant miasm within every individual. This will unfortunately place the book in a position of disagreement with other authors whose miasmatic understanding varies from this, but differing opinions are a healthy sign of a thinking profession and should be viewed as such.

3. **References outside of Homoeopathy.** I have drawn many thoughts and opinions for the extension of this miasmatic model from areas outside of Homoeopathy. These areas include Christianity, Buddhism, the Kabbalah, traditional shamanism, Rosicrucian mysticism, psychology and quantum physics. Aspects of all of these have helped formulate a comprehensive theoretical model that defines a miasm.

4. **Facial feature recognition.** It needs to be clarified that when I talk of reading a face or understanding facial features as miasmatic indicators, I am not referring to either physiognomy or Siang mien. Both of these arts recognise individual facial features as external guides to internal character traits. Therefore both systems claim a degree of emotional diagnosis that is not undertaken

here. I have read many of their texts and have become acquainted with both systems during the research of this book, but in both cases I have found them inappropriate for our specialised Homoeopathic needs. It soon became apparent that the best way to develop a model that specifically catered for the needs of the Homoeopathic profession was to start the whole model from scratch. Therefore any crossover information is purely coincidental. Miasmatic prescribing through facial feature recognition gives a practitioner firm footing and confidence to place their patients into a miasmatic group, it does not define character.

With all these points in mind, I present to you my understanding of the miasms.

ACKNOWLEDGEMENTS
(Homeopathic Facial Analysis 2006)

To all who have been involved in this project and to those who support facial analysis, I wish to extend my deepest and most sincere heartfeltthanks.

To practitioners both local and international prepared to try facial analysis. I appreciate your enthusiasm and willingness to inform me of your successes, it has been a great encouragement and I am thrilled it has such supporters.

To my patients and students, especially those who once again answered the call to contribute by allowing me to use their features so others can learn.

To all my children for their cooperation and contribution to this book, thanks for your patience, your interest and your belief in facial analysis, your support is invaluable and I love you all dearly.

To my mother and extended family, for allowing their faces to be scrutinized, analysed and publicized just to help us out, thanks to you all.

To Allan for his publishing expertise and help once again.

To my homoeopathic teacher Denise, who was overlooked in the acknowledgements in *Appearance and Circumstance* .

To Heather Betts who has been nothing short of a Godsend. Heathers talent and commitment is responsible for all the illustrations in this book. Without Heather, this book would be nothing more than a good idea. Many people, patients and practitioners alike will benefit due to effort and skill.

Finally, to my wife Louise, the third party in the sleepless trio that put this book together. Her contribution to the book as well as to facial analysis as a system has been extensive. Facial analysis as a system would not exist if it was not for Louise and that is the plain and simple truth. Her contributions include the addition of certain facial features, help in the development of its theory and formulating an evaluation process to categorize remedies. Louise is responsible for many of the methods and remedies other practitioners using facial analysis put into practice every day. It may be my name on the cover but it is not a one-man show and Louise has achieved all this while running a family, a clinic and a college. It is my sincere hope that she finds pride in this achievement. From our family and from me- we love you.

CONTENTS

Homeopathic Facial Analysis 2006

INTRODUCTION
(Homeopathic Facial Analysis 2006)

It has been four years since *Appearance and Circumstance* was written and the system of facial analysis continues to evolve. Clearer facial features, better case taking and repertorising techniques, as well as a comprehensive understanding of homeopathic philosophy has shaped a complete picture of what miasms are and how they work.

With hindsight, *Appearance and Circumstance* is a better introductory book into the theory of facial analysis and miasms than it is an actual training manual. This second book is dedicated entirely to practical facial analysis, in an attempt to remedy any of the shortfalls found in *Appearance and Circumstance* .

One of the major challenges of facial analysis is defining normal limits. When does a nose become wide or a bridge indented? What does a cleft in the chin actually mean? While many have found the verbal definitions and photos in *Appearance and Circumstance* to be adequate, others require more visual parameters. In this book, every effort has been made to ensure each facial feature is as clearly defined as possible, making the system easier to use. Once mastered facial analysis offers a solid foundation for prescribing, and rewards homoeopaths prepared to give it time and practice with a consistency of success generally reserved to highly experienced practitioners.

Facial analysis is based on a perfect quality and knowledge of nature and while it still requires expertise and finesse, it does not rely on subjective interpretation and that is its greatest strength. The weakness of subjective analysis is due to the fact that the range of human thought and emotion is limitless and beyond our verbal capacity to express it. Put simply, there are more experiences and feelings than there are words to describe them, therefore we have to squeeze experience into the barriers imposed by vocabulary.

Sadness for example is felt in numerous forms and degrees, but it is still called sadness by those who endure it. We often choose sadness as a word to best describe how we feel because there are so few available alternatives.

Words convey thoughts and emotions from one mind to another; they attempt to make others understand what we are thinking and feeling, words try to make another person understand what its like to be us. However, for language to be effective it must be basic, because only the basic can be understood by all. Language that inhibits communication is useless if the person we intend the words for fail to recognize them. For words to be useful, the thoughts or feelings they represent must be easily understood. Therefore, the most effective words to express emotions are those most commonly understood. Our problem is that common does not individualize. Therefore, we can never fully understand another persons experience via language because of the need to sacrifice the distinctive for the familiar. A system based entirely on subjective sensation and feeling walks a tight-rope. Boenninghausen recognized this over a century ago which is why he preferred generals over mentals, not because they are better per se, but because they are less subjective and therefore more reliable. Even Hahnemann, although he placed a great deal of emphasis on the mentals did so always in conjunction with the generals.

The law of similars is based on a faith in nature, follow her lead and things will fall into place, analyze without faith and you run the risk of intellectualizing yourself out of the natural and into a man-made theory based more on supposition than on fact. This was homeopathy's criticism of allopathy. Like the great homeopaths of old, our aim is to work with nature not to reinterpret it. Facial analysis is nature at work. Hahnemann understood that nature is all-knowing and that we are not. Hahnemann surrendered himself to nature and used signs and symptoms as a guide to health rather than an enemy to eradicate. By following nature's lead Hahnemann developed the most sophisticated medical system the world has ever known.

Homeopathy developed from what Hahnemann saw. He put speculation aside and used what existed as his guide to the truth. He knew that two similar diseases could not exist in the same body at the same time because nature told him so. He accepted it as fact and utilized it.

Homoeopathy proved itself in the acute diseases. Typhus, cholera, smallpox, and scarlet fever, all had their sting cut short thanks to Hahnemann. In chronic disease however, his approach needed to differ. Hahnemann acknowledged that he could treat acute disease successfully, but failed when it came to treating the predisposition to disease. We all know the story of his unflagging effort to find a solution to this problem as well as his steadfast belief in the correctness of the miasm theory and yet even now chronic disease continues to create uncertainty.

It would be fair to say that on an historical timeline homoeopathy reached its greatest height during the period when many homoeopathic doctors were using it for acute diseases and ailments. Its relatively recent demise is both fractured and complicated and it is not just because the A.M.A declared war on us and didn't fight fair, that it far too simplistic. I am not saying that this was not a factor, as far as hurdles go, having the A.M.A against you is a 'big one' in anyone's language, but nothing is learned if we do not accept at least some of the responsibility.

As time progressed, homoeopathy's role has moved from the acute to the chronic especially for non-medical homoeopaths. The trouble is, without medical training the base line of diagnosis has disappeared. I understand that a homoeopath should never start with pathology yet at the same time 'genus epidemicus' was invaluable and consistently used.

Unfortunately, in chronic disease genus epidemicus does not apply and there is a good reason for this. Genus epidemicus is applicable in acute disease only because acute disease is more about the virus or bacteria and its impact on the individual than on the individual themselves. This is not the case with chronic disease because chronic disease is 'man- made' and therefore any viruses or bacteria that go along with the diagnosis do so as a consequence not as a cause. Chronic disease is about the person who has the disease - acute is a mixture of impact and resistance.

It is my belief that part of the reason homoeopathy is in its current depleted state is because chronic disease remains elusive and difficult to alleviate. Hahnemann knew the rules that had to be applied – work out the miasm according to psora, sycosis and syphilis then select the best remedy that fits both the totality of symptoms as well as the miasm, the rest should take care of itself. Yet Hahnemann's own records show that while he knew what to do in theory, the practical application of this theory remained troublesome.

Facial analysis overcomes the previous difficulties of chronic disease and brings homoeopathy into the position Hahnemann envisaged. I believe, facial analysis in chronic disease is the completion of Hahnemann's work.

'Nature always knows best' has always been homoeopathy's creed, facial analysis is an extension of this.

PUBLISHER'S NOTE

Miasms remain a topic of controversy in homeopathy and on the majority of occasions views are different and varied. What is important for a theory or explanation is its practical application. As far as understanding miasms is concerned, the theory or method needs to have criterions which are less subjective, are quantifiable or measurable and therefore more reliable. The method of Homeopathic Facial Analysis (HFA) by Grant Bentley is very much on these lines. HFA is a research project of more than ten years, tested clinically worldwide and successful feedback has been received regarding its application.

What Grant says is that prescribing solely on personality types is a way which can be very successful at times and can lead to failures at times. The reason stated is very right that all people will not fit into the personality types at all times. People or remedies go through phases and they might not be in the phase you know that drug as. What is suggested is to prescribe on remedy criterion and miasm combined so the choice of medicine is reduced and it also checks the accuracy of the prescription at a certain level.

The intention of facial analysis is to give the practitioner a way to classify the patient into a miasmatic group and therefore the choice of remedy is reduced and accuracy of the prescriptions are increased. The steps to applying facial analysis are objective criterions and that is the greatest strength of this method.

We are happy to bring this work which has been very successful in the west and hope that it is used and applied by the practitioners in Asia and thus help in giving a newer understanding to miasms and their application. We are thankful to Grant and Louise for they agreed to bring this work to this part of the world through us and hope it's received with as much enthusiasm as we believe it deserves.

- Kuldeep Jain, CEO

CONTENTS

PART ONE
MIASMS

The miasms are like enemies entrenched.

- J H Allen

CHAPTER 1

Methodology

Try to master this: Diseases must not be looked upon from a few symptoms that the patient may possess but from all the symptoms that the whole human race brings out. It is just as improper to look upon psora from a few symptoms as it is to look upon a remedy from a few symptoms. Just as you see the image of a remedy from all the symptoms, including the peculiar symptoms, so psora must be considered from its characteristics, the features that constitute psora. Remedies are adjusted as to appearance; the appearances of the remedy expressed in symptoms must be adjusted to the appearances of the diseases expressed in symptoms. When you have finished psora, take up sycosis, and spend much time in gathering together all the symptoms that sycotic patients have felt, all the suffering and all the ultimates. Group them as one, and look upon them as one miasm. Then go to the Materia Medica again and make an anamnesis. Take each symptom and place opposite it all the remedies that have produced that symptom. You can readily see that the remedies that run through most strongly will be anti-sycotic remedies, i.e., the remedies that have the essentials of the disease or the nature of sycosis in them.

- J.T. Kent

Whilst I stated in the introduction that I am unsure as to how the miasmatic identification process first began, I can recall a few years ago, pondering on whether or not down-turned eyes could be a distinguishing feature of psora? I had recently treated some patients who had responded extremely well to Pulsatilla and was at that time wondering if this appearance could be an external manifestation of Pulsatilla as a remedy as two of my three Pulsatilla patients had this facial feature. However after this I changed track and began wondering if rather than belonging to Pulsatilla, could down-turned eyes belong to the broader category of psora? If this was so, then other miasms would also have signature features. Soon I had another psoric patient that responded well, and they too had down-turned eyes. Could it be that certain facial features belong to specific miasmatic groups? Knowing that there is nothing new under the sun I began to search for comments on the subject by other homoeopaths either past or present.

I was not expecting to find a comprehensive study, but if this thought process was credible there should be some previous reference to it. The first was found in J H Allen's book *The Chronic Miasms and Pseudo-Psora* of the most universally respected and comprehensive books ever written on the subject of miasms, it is full of details, descriptions and examples that highlight the validity of facial features as an indicative basis in which to identify a particular miasm. I reached a conclusion; miasms exert their influence just as comprehensively on the outside as they do on the inside, it simply cannot be any other way. It is not possible that one's outside appearance can bear an entirely different relationship to the miasmatic/genetic factors that formulated it. Every facet of our lives is governed by our genes, including our appearance; our miasm influences our genes, so our miasm can be depicted by our appearance.

As a student I was taught that a skin rash is the outward manifestation of some inner turmoil, and yet for some reason the concept that a miasm could influence, let alone determine someone's appearance seemed farfetched. It is now implausible for it to be any other way. The underlying dominant miasm in each and every one of us is as plain as the nose, mouth, eyes and everything else on our face.

At this point I believe it prudent to highlight one of the many examples from J H Allen.

How generally we see the landmarks of one of these chronic miasms stamped upon the organism. We see it in every feature and every physiological process; in the shape and contour of the body; upon the visual expression, the face, nose, lips, ears, mouth, upon the hair, its growth, lustre and general beauty or lack of it. We see it upon the skin in its colour or shadings, its local temperature, yes, we can tell the miasm often by a touch, by that response in our very inner being, the mental, the moral, even the spiritual, give us responses of its presence and of its influence.

Allen leaves us in no doubt of his belief that a miasm imparts an indelible imprint on the organism. He reasons that the miasm is so much a part of genetic material that it can alter us in accordance with its own unique but destructive form. As a consequence, the dividing line between miasm and DNA erodes into non-existence as one is deemed an expression of the other. Hence for this model, miasmatic influence and genetic predisposition are recognised as interchangeable terms.

Hints regarding miasmatic facial features occur not just in Allen's book, but throughout Roberts' *Art and Principles of Cure by Homoeopathy* For example, in Chapter 23, regarding psora he writes:

Psora alone never causes structural changes, and the psoric head is normal in size and contour. The hair and scalp are dry, rarely perspiring; the hair is lustreless and so dry that it cannot be combed without wetting the comb. The hair falls out after an illness. It becomes gray too early, or white in spots; it breaks and the ends split. [And again in the same chapter] The shape of the psoric face is that of an inverted pyramid ... The lips are red, often red to bluish, parched and dry.

In reference to syphilis Roberts writes:

In the mouth we find the characteristic tell-tale of the syphilitic taint, even though the child may appear well otherwise. Pathological and structural changes take place in the dental arch and the teeth come through deformed, irregular in shape and irregular in order of eruption. The teeth often decay before they are entirely through the gums ...The appearance of people suffering from the syphilitic stigma often tells the story at a glance, for we observe that the head is large and bulging, the hair is moist, gluey, greasy ...

Reference regarding appearance is also found in more recent works from authors such as Donald Foubister:

My interest in Carcinosin was aroused by a chance experience: that of having in the out-patient department simultaneously two children born of mothers who were, during the pregnancy, suffering from cancer of the breast. These children presented a remarkably similar appearance, having blue sclerotics, a cafe au lait complexion and numerous moles.

Further on following the same line of inquiry he writes:

It soon became apparent that children of what we came to regard as the *"Carcinosin appearance" did not show the kind of family history we had almost expected to find. In many instances there was a strong family history of cancer, but in others there was a strong family history of tuberculosis, of diabetes and pernicious anaemia, or a combination of all these more strongly represented than in the average family...*

Although he does go on to highlight that more research is needed into the area of distinguishing characteristics, Foubister does affirm his belief in an "appearance trend".

It is clear that practitioners like Foubister, Roberts and Allen believe that far more than just pathology is influenced by the miasms. They, along with many other authors, past and present, go further than just disease outcomes when describing what a miasm is. These authors believe an individual's whole demeanor and psychology is moulded by their dominating miasm. Where both Allen and Roberts differ from other writers on the subject, is in the importance they place on physical appearance as miasmatic indicators.

This book is a continuation of the theme and work that originated with these two great homoeopaths.

A frequently asked question is: "Why such a focus on the face? Surely a miasm should exhibit its influence everywhere on the body, height or weight or hair colouring." And this is absolutely true, the miasms influence everything including all of the above; in reality a practitioner should be able to tell the dominant miasm from a patient's toenail if they had the knowledge of how to do it, but the face has been chosen as the most accurate transmitter of miasmatic information for two primary reasons:

1. The face can be easily examined. Unlike a toenail, the face is exposed and can be viewed directly by the practitioner during the consultation, indeed good eye contact and facial response is expected during a homoeopathic consultation, anything less and it could be perceived by the patient that the practitioner is uninterested. Hence the face can be examined openly and at length.

The face is expressive and exposed; it is also one of the only body parts that an outsider is allowed to continually look at without disturbing custom and social etiquette.

2. The face is by far our most characteristic and expressive feature, it expresses every emotion we have, the moment we have it. Or to the contrary, it may remain poker faced when it should be expressive; either way the face speaks volumes in regards to personality and position. As with most things, it's the extremes that pose the greatest challenge. In the case of the face, it is the extreme ends of age, the very young or the very old, that are always the most difficult to determine. But for most of our patients it is true to say that the face offers us the best observable account of their genetic inheritance combined with their life experience. Both are etched into the face just waiting to be examined. Genetic/ miasmatic inheritance will be evident in the bone structure and design of the face, while their life experience shows itself through the lines and contours. Because the face has a varied and extensive musculature, it will readily contort itself in accordance to the emotions we feel. A facial expression is a reactive observable response designed to convey the internal emotion being experienced. Just as a body builder regularly works on a particular muscle group to achieve a distinct shape, so the muscles of our face also become sculpted and developed. Consequently they will take on the corresponding shape formed by the exercise/emotion they perform most regularly. In short we are responsible for the tired or angry or worried countenance that we bear. Only the face chronicles with such precision an individual's life potential and their outcomes. No other area of the body allows us an insight into capability and condition like that provided by the face.

In earlier times when there was less reliance on technology

and a greater reliance on observation, practitioners, both homoeopathic and allopathic, noticed reproducible trends that not only ran through families but often ran through sufferers of a particular disease. Hahnemann was the greatest and most well known observer of pathological trends and this skill is how the whole concept of the miasms started their life. But he was not the only person to notice distinctive patterns left behind by specific diseases. The ongoing hereditary ramifications of syphilis were not just recognised by Hahnemann alone, indeed acknowledgement of this trend fathered the now almost lost discipline of syphilology. Part of this medical specialisation was heredosyphilis – the study of the observable familial traits to indicate that syphilis had visited a family.

In his book titled *Modern Clinical Syphilology* written in 1926, doctor and author John H Stokes comments about heredosyphilis in babies and highlights the importance of structural recognition. The clinical picture he writes, "will include snuffles, causeless crying and screaming" and "a café au lait colouring...As the patient gets older they may display features like a saddle across the nose and wide separation of the eyes". Any or all of these signs alerted an astute physician to the possibility of syphilitic infection. Blood tests were then taken and a positive or negative infection decision was made. However these physicians were looking for the actual disease of syphilis and with a failure to accept the theory of latency, clinical tests would be forever highlighting the "spurious" nature of facial feature recognition; hence it was never highly regarded as a therapeutic tool and as a consequence remained a dormant and undeveloped application.

Homoeopaths, however, understand the importance of latency and predisposition. We understand that the failure of a particular disease to manifest physically does not mean freedom from its miasmatic influence. We understand as Donald Foubister highlighted, that there are other possible disease results, all of which are understandable and predictable if one just substitutes the words "trend" or "possibility" for "specific outcomes or consequence". What is important is to understand that the same facial features that indicated the presence of syphilis in John H Stokes's day are just as valid today. These features are as common and distinctive now as they were then. What has been lost is our ability to recognise and interpret them.

In the past, for allopaths, "pathological facial features" such as the ones just described indicated the possibility of syphilis, for present day homoeopaths who understand predisposition, these facial features still indicate the possibility of syphilis, not as a disease but as a miasm.

The course of action now was to concentrate on cataloguing a patient's salient features and deciding to which miasmatic family each patient belonged; in that way a comprehensive dossier could be built for each miasmatic group.

Before I explain how the information was gathered, I wish to emphasise one important point: as few previous works in this field exist, much of the data had to be gathered and expanded upon through successful clinical cases. Validation of all relevant information has taken place via the "trend spotting" method only clinical practice can provide. Everything in this book in regards to themes and facial features has been arrived at via this manner, no provings have been conducted. When a patient had a good constitutional result, that is, a significant improvement in their health, energy and happiness, their circumstances had changed for the better and a major amelioration in the general features of the case occurred, then and only then would that patient be considered appropriate to learn from.

In order to gain the information needed clinically, two important benchmarks were laid down:

1. All the consultations and prescriptions to be considered must be from a constitutional prescription, not organic. The definition of the two differing approaches being, constitutional prescribing priorities mental outlook, emotional responses and all the relevant generals of a case without concentration on pathology, whilst an organic prescription satisfies itself by directing its focus on the nature of the presenting complaint or by centering on the most primary organ under stress.

2. There had to be obvious physical pathology in every case under consideration by which an accurate measure as to the success of the remedy could be made. Only those who responded both mentally and physically were further analysed in reference to their backgrounds, heredity and physical makeup.

This second point is vital as experience shows that patients can feel better in themselves while pathology can remain untouched. Functional and structural pathology are vital indicators of positive change. Patients will often remark how they feel "better already" before the remedy is even given but this does not necessarily flow on to actual physical change. Kent in his writings suggests that once the patient feels better in themselves, the rest will automatically fall into place. But I am going to be impertinent and suggest that physical symptoms should reduce in conjunction with and at the same corresponding level to the mental symptoms of the case. Oftentimes patients get to release or come face to face with emotions and beliefs that have evaded or tormented them for years, in some cases for a whole lifetime. The weight that is lifted from their shoulders before any medicine has even been given cannot be overestimated, but that lifted weight will rarely change structural pathology, only the appropriate homoeopathic remedy can take it that one step further.

In regards to taking down the heredity details, the formula was uncomplicated, merely a few simple questions regarding parents and grandparents, a brief health history – cause of death and their age when they died, from both sides of the family. If a patient could take their lineage further that would be a bonus, but few could, in fact most patients were stumbling when it came to grandparents let alone going any further.

Once a case was deemed successful, the next step was to photograph the patient. This was done on a digital camera and transferred to computer for closer scrutiny. From here, the major "stand out" features were identified and allocated to their appropriate miasm. The photograph of a patient should be examined on a computer screen rather than viewing the patient's actual face as digital photographs allow you to highlight and zoom in on certain features, which would otherwise be too invasive and confrontational.

In the beginning, the most important cases were those in which a remedy from an unmistakable miasmatic group was successful, so results from remedies like Sulphur or Mercury or Thuja, etc., became of prime importance. Establishing a base line of this type is important as it forms a platform on which more lateral concepts can be experimented with.

Step two in the examination process was to collate all the successful Thuja and Medorrhinum and Sepia cases into one sycotic file and after a sufficient quantity of photographs had been gained, patient's faces were closely examined in relation to each other. Here all Sulphur and Psorinum cases were compared, all Mercury and Aurum, etc.

This process allows the distinctive facial features that belong to each particular miasm to emerge. For example, slightly protruding or exophthalmic eyes began to surface as a sycotic feature, showing itself in a number of patients who had responded well to sycotic remedies. This process uncovers commonality rather than individuality. Therefore if exophthalmic eyes are seen in both Medorrhinum and Thuja patients, then exophthalmic or protruding eyes become an observable clinical sign as to the presence of sycosis. This observation is clinically tested against a number of patients before confirmation is given. Hence the process of facial feature identification begins when a characteristic facial feature shows itself enough times in patients who have responded to remedies belonging to the same miasmatic family.

While some patients with exophthalmic eyes also showed other quite observable sycotic characteristics, others displayed features already classified into other miasmatic groups. For a while I was toying with the idea that two miasms could share the same facial feature, for example a patient who presented with the exophthalmic eyes of sycosis but also had the domed or curved forehead of syphilis could still be fully sycotic if a bulging forehead was sycotic as well as syphilitic. The range of possible explanations includes:

1. Exophthalmic eyes belonged to both sycosis and syphilis.

2. A bulging or domed shaped forehead may belong to both sycosis and syphilis.

3. A dome-shaped or curved forehead was never part of syphilis in the first place, it had been sycotic all along.

4. Exophthalmic eyes had never been sycotic they should have been placed in the syphilitic group.

I also postulated as to whether a layers type approach should be adopted as it provided an obvious solution. This means that the patient's facial features indicate that both the syphilitic and sycotic miasms are present and that perhaps remedies from both miasms will be needed alternately throughout the management of the case.

But patients with exophthalmic eyes and other trademark sycotic features, had responded exceptionally well to sycotic remedies alone without any alternation. The solution lay in rethinking and remodelling the number of miasms that conventional homoeopathic literature claims exist. If one stays with the traditional notion of four major miasms, five if cancer is included, then the problem becomes almost insurmountable, but when this number was extended, the explanation became clear.

As with all things homoeopathic, the answer lay inside the pages of the *Organon*

Hahnemann himself saw that two dissimilar chronic diseases could co-exist forming a chronic disease complex with its own unique makeup and nature. In Aphorism Forty he writes: "Or the new disease, after having long acted on the organism, at length joins the old one that is dissimilar to it and forms with it a complex disease." Hence, two chronic diseases or miasms, provided they are of equal strength (otherwise the stronger will repel the weaker) can join together to make a separate, combined or complex miasm.

The basis of all chronic disease, according to Hahnemann, belonged to infection by one of the chronic miasms. As can be seen in *The Genius of Homoeopathy* by Stuart Close (quoting Hahnemann):

If we deduct all chronic affections, ailments and diseases that depend on a persistent unhealthy mode of living, as also those innumerable medicinal maladies caused by the irrational, persistent, harassing and pernicious treatment of diseases often only of trivial character by physicians of the old school, all the remainder, without exception, result from the development of these three chronic miasms, internal syphilis, internal sycosis, but chiefly and in infinitely greater proportion, internal psora, each of which was already in possession of the whole organism ...

All chronic illness has its foundation in the miasms, each miasm will alter the body in its own inimitable fashion, but two dissimilar miasms can join together to form another miasm just as unique. These miasms come from and retain many of the qualities of their parent miasms yet exhibit an idiosyncratic flavour.

Many books, Allen's in particular, give numerous accounts of a sycosyphilitic or sycopsoric miasm at work. References to "complex miasms" may also be found in more modern texts on the subject such as *Miasmatic Diagnosis* by Subrata Banerjea, in which clinical details of the "psorasycotic" are discussed.

The explanation as to why some patients show signs of sycosis as well as signs of syphilis is because they contain elements of both. Many of these perplexing patients belonged to a complex group, they were not sycotic or syphilitic they were sycosyphilitic. I did not understand until much later that single miasmatic facial features do not indicate an equal footing of the particular miasm they represent. Hence one syphilitic feature amongst six other sycotic facial features does not make a patient syco-syphilitic – a six to one ratio only serves to show the dominance of sycosis.

We are what we think. All that we are arises with our thoughts. With our thoughts, we make the world.

- Buddha

CHAPTER 2

What is a Miasm?

All cases present early mental symptoms, and there is always a trail of symptoms, mental and nervous, until the development of tuberculosis is well established; then the mental symptoms disappear, and in most cases there has been an absence of mental symptoms for a period before the beginning of the deposits. This leads to the opinion that there is in nearly all cases a predisposition to tuberculosis, and it is this predisposition that is inherited. If this is absent, protection is quite positive.

- J.T. Kent

Defining the exact nature of a miasm is a task more difficult than it may at first seem. No wonder there is confusion in applying the miasms clinically when there seem to be so many different definitions of what they actually are. It is often presumed that Hahnemann's belief about the miasms is the same as Kent's or Roberts's, but this is not the case. What's more, the differences between them can be quite remarkable and those differences have an enormous impact on the way each clinical practice is conducted. Defining a miasm is of the utmost importance as each differing definition brings with it its own therapeutic process and system based on its interpretation, and these different understandings are not as interchangeable or complementary as one might think. Indeed in some circumstances, the acceptance of one miasmatic viewpoint may preclude the belief in another as they are so different.

Hahnemann believed that miasms arose from organic infective agents like syphilis or leprosy which, when combined with medical mismanagement and suppressive treatments served to drive the localised disease inwards where it then became systemic and permeated every cell in the body, tormenting its sufferer until the end of their days. This previously localised disease became internalised when inappropriate medical treatments such as salves for the scabies eruption or cauterisation of a syphilitic chancre prevented the body collecting all the internal poisons into one localised spot or area. If the body's attempt at capturing the poison is prevented, Hahnemann asserted that the disease became liberated from its prison and escaped into any or all of the internal areas of the body it could occupy. The sufferer is now entirely infected and a miasm has been formed. A miasm then is a disease that has overcome the body's defences and is unable to be removed; it is now free to impart its influence.

Hahnemann believed two different chronic diseases/miasms of equal strength could exist in the same body at the same time, but one of two outcomes would occur

1. Two miasms would cohabit the same body each occupying the body system or area best suited to it and leaving the other miasm alone to do the same.

2. The two different chronic diseases would join together to form a complex disease.

In summary, Hahnemann's view of a miasm is one where a contagious infection has been medically mismanaged and in consequence becomes a systemic illness that permeates the entire physical body to such an extent that the disease imprint can now be genetically transferred from one generation to the next.

It is often stated, that Kent was a strict Hahnemannian, following exactly the laws and principles laid down by Hahnemann; in fact no one states this fact more often than James Tyler Kent himself, but the truth is Kent often deviated from Hahnemann and frequently added his own flavour. One of the areas in which he did this is the miasms. Hahnemann not only believed that the miasms were of microbial origin he also believed that psora was so contagious that *nearly* everybody had it. Kent however introduced a different variation on the subject:

Psora is the underlying cause, and is the primitive or primary disorder of the human race. It is a disordered state of the internal economy of the human race. This state expresses itself in the forms of the varying chronic diseases, or chronic manifestations. If the human race had remained in a state of perfect order, psora could not have existed. The susceptibility to psora opens out a question altogether too broad to study among the sciences in a medical college. It is altogether too extensive, for it goes to the very primitive wrong of the human race, the very first sickness of the human race, that is the spiritual sickness, from which first state the race progressed into what may be called the true susceptibility to psora, which in turn laid the foundation for other diseases. If we regard psora as synonymous with itch, we fail to understand, and fail to express thereby, anything like the original intention of Hahnemann. The itch is commonly supposed to be a limited thing, something superficial, caused by a little tiny bit of a mite that is supposed to have life, and when the little itch mite is destroyed the cause of itch is said to have been removed. What a folly!

From this we can derive three very important facts regarding Kent's personal definition of a miasm.

1. He regards the idea that psora is indistinguishable from and originated from scabies to be "folly".

2. Kent is clearly addressing everyone when he uses terms like the human race. Hence he considers everyone to be psoric.

3. Kent regards the whole topic of the miasms beyond the scope of medicine, as the roots of psora extend beyond the physical into the metaphysical. They are, as he points out, of "spiritual" origin and certainly not bacterial.

Kent in relation to psora believed that the true underlying miasm is the evil or sin that is within us.

Hence this state, the state of the human mind and the state of the human body, is a state of susceptibility to disease from willing evils, from thinking that which is false and making life one continuous heredity of false things, and so this form of disease, psora, is but an outward manifestation of that which is prior in man. It was not due to actions of the body, as we find syphilis and sycosis to be, but due to an influx from a state, which progressed and established itself upon the earth, until we can see it as but the outward manifestations of man's very nature.

All the physical psoric symptoms we see are the predictable consequences and manifestations of incorrect thinking. According to Kent we are all caught in an addiction of negativity, a sin as Kent prefers to put it, and because of its hold on us we comply with its wishes habitually. Every life is dominated by its craving and all emotional and physical weaknesses exist because of it. We are all slaves to the fears and insecurities the miasms impart to us, in fact everything that takes away our freedom to be who we really want to be, the "I'm not good enough", that creeps in with every plan, the "I'm different", "worse", "less capable", "misunderstood", etc., each one of these negative self-images, along with a veritable library of others is what Kent referred to when he spoke of the true essence or understanding of the nature of psora.

Dr Ortega in the introduction to his book on the miasms writes:

When we come to understand in all their amplitude the meaning of the terms psora, sycosis and syphilis – in the far-reaching definition given them by Hahnemann – we will have answers to all the questions which can be formulated in medicine and biology. This will enable us to deduce everything relating to man's conduct and the expression of his being... Here and now we must warn against even beginning to read these pages with a concept of illness, especially chronic illness or miasm, as something material which is encrusted onto, or added to, the complex functioning of the human entity. Instead, it should be seen as a manner of being of this entity, one state of existence out of the many which can be adopted or produced by this invisible entity... An understanding of the miasmatic, is in our judgement, the ultimate concern of the physician, because it involves nothing less than a maximum understanding of the human, both with respect to the qualities which lead him to persist and to realize his full potential, and with respect to those defects which hinder him...

My definition of a miasm is in harmony with this; miasms are a non-contagious spiritual anomaly present in every human being that may manifest in various forms but always contain the same underlying themes together with the universal result of inhibition, fear and hatred. It is my intention to show that miasms are the homoeopathic equivalent of Buddhism's ego and Christianity's devil. Miasms are the defects and irregularities present in each and every one of us from birth. They influence who we think we are, what we think we like to do and who we think we relate to. They are the sum total of our fears and phobias. They do not contribute anything of positive value. They are inhibitors that serve no other purpose than to place doubt where none should exist. It is true that some negative emotions have a justifiable origin. For example, not all guilt is inappropriate, sometimes it is a protest from a higher consciousness telling us to desist from our current course of action or else we and others will suffer. If that suffering should already be occurring, guilt is needed to remind us of what actions led us down this path so they are not repeated. But there is also unjustifiable guilt, a continuous nagging that makes a person feel responsible for everything that occurs around them and encourages self-blame and torment. Fear has a legitimate and valuable place, it serves as a great protector, but continuous fear only leads to a life unlived, it dominates choice of surroundings and choice of partner, it can dominate decision-making and a whole life can be designed around it or to achieve relief from it. Whether one lives a life dominated by one's miasmatic passions or a life dedicated to avoiding them the result is still the same – the miasm is dictating the terms.

Miasmatic understanding for me started with a personal attempt to try and come to terms with a subject that for the most part was confusing and academic. In time I came to understand that the miasms were far more than potential disease patterns, and the model began to show that psychological outlooks always accompany chronic disease. While this is not new or exclusive to homoeopathy it is still enthralling to see it in action. What is new, however, is that facial features can give an accurate account of the most prevalent miasm in a person, and in addition each miasm has a predictable psychological theme. From a patient's appearance it is now possible for a practitioner to determine what miasm is dominant and as such, understand the most likely prime motivating factors in their life. I now understand why some people place extreme importance on things that others will hold in contempt. A study into the miasms will show that in the timeless argument of nature verses nurture, nature wins hands down. Depression, fear, even a calm rational attitude under pressure owe their existence to an instinctive stress response dictated by the miasm. The miasms are the pre-existent state that Kent spoke of, this "thing" that comes before all others of which everything else is either an expression or consequence. Thought always precedes the action; the will always comes before the outcome.

Everything and everyone has an energy into which the physical will soon manifest. Ancient mystics spoke in terms of how each person, thing and event that happens here on earth, has already occurred in the higher planes. Energy comes first and once in place becomes increasingly dense until the physical takes form. Energy means circumstances are already in motion before the thought has even occurred. An event like a body merely grows into the space provided by the pattern that preceded it.

As practitioners we are privy to very personal information, details of events and secrets many thought they would take to the grave. From this privileged vantage point we are able to see how events continually repeat themselves. Some people know nothing but drama in their lives, others nothing but love. With some, a random violent act is no great surprise while to someone else it is something that happens to others. Everyone has an energy about them that will attract similar energies into their life and this energy can manifest as a person, disease or event. After the appropriate remedy circumstances begin to change, jobs begin to be offered to individuals who had been unemployed, bad relationships end so good relationships can begin.

Clinical experience has shown this truth so many times, that now during a followup consultation, no matter how much a person may claim to be better, if negative circumstances continue to occur I will disregard my previous prescription and search out a new and better one. None of this is a conscious decision, of course, no one wakes up in the morning and contemplates how they can make their life worse, but it is vital to understand at a subconscious or energetic level that anything or event that occurs continuously is most assuredly coming from the energy of that person. This patterning determines life events, it does not occur the other way around; once the miasms are fully understood a predictability can be seen running through all these random events. This is not a fatalist attitude, miasmatic patterning can be changed, but it takes either a major lifestyle or mindset change. By far the easiest way to achieve this change is by the right homoeopathic remedy.

The same can be said about physical pathology; potential always precedes outcome. No one can exceed their genetic potential either physically or intellectually, one can live up to it but to exceed it is to venture beyond design and that is simply impossible. Whether a person's latent potential fulfils itself is up to the free will of the individual.

An energy surrounds each and every one of us and this energy influences the way we feel about ourselves and the events that occur in our life, indeed listening to the sequence of events in a patient's life is often the best way to determine the type of energy that exists around them. Listen to their choice of words, recognise the type of people they draw towards them, the type of work they do, the hobbies they have, hear about the worst things that have happened to them and the "accidents" that have befallen them, for there will be a pattern, and "pattern" is just another name for miasm. This pattern is discernible, inherited and treatable.

We are all going to reach our destination one way or the other, either we will apply experience and wisdom to make our transition or else life will take control and teach us through experience. However, as with Hering's law, each time a symptom/lesson is driven into the system or ignored, it is replaced by new symptoms or events more serious and dramatic than the one that preceded it. The purpose of a remedy is to help experience become wisdom as quickly and easily as possible; in this way the same mistakes do not need to be repeated over and over again, the remedy can give insight, enabling an individual to break patterns and to take charge of their life. Perhaps it will assist them to accept what is, either way it will do what is most required for the benefit of that person.

What is the difference between miasms and karma? The short answer is, there is no difference at all. Miasmatic knowledge is nothing more than the age-old laws of karma with a medicinal application.

I understand that a conclusion such as this regarding the miasms takes it out of the realm of science, and some homoeopaths will feel uncomfortable with that, but the truth is, I have had these conclusions forced upon me. I have not devised a model to fit a pre-existing belief. Some homoeopaths want to ally themselves with scientific medicine and that is their prerogative, some take it further and have made an incorporation with allopathy their mission. Homoeopathy, rightly so, should be taken seriously and it should be validated, it is a successful integrated system that changes lives for the better, but it does not need outside validation; only the homoeopathic profession itself can bestow the credibility it deserves.

My personal opinion is that homoeopathy is a reproducible medical miracle, it is not an allopathic analogue. What homoeopathy offers is outside the realms of allopathy, its whole philosophical belief system is so profound and distinct that the two systems simply cannot "complement" one another. Both parties should leave well enough alone and be content. We should be proud and uncompromising about who we are. Reread Hahnemann or Kent or Roberts, they all knew that homoeopathy is a separate and unique system and they defended that difference with all their energy. They knew a fact that we sometimes overlook; doctors do not make the best homoeopaths, nor do psychologists or naturopaths, homoeopaths make the best homoeopaths. Kent, for example, knew all too well that homoeopathy transcended standard medical beliefs and methods, he grasped very quickly there was far more to this new system than the nuts and bolts mechanics of "old school" thinking.

I have stated that karma and the miasms are interchangeable aspects of one another, but this is only in respect to the law of similars. Karma is the product of countless lifetimes; some consider it a debt, others more a lesson, while others consider it a resolution. I don't know if the miasms are the same as this, I'm not even sure if I believe in past lives the more I begin to understand about cellular memory, but where karma and the miasms do blend is in the understanding that everything has its prior cause. Karma means that what you put out, you will have returned; not revenge, just logic. In this way each individual becomes their own moral judge to hand down their own sentences until we are forced to address ourselves. Buddhism calls it karma, science calls this cause and effect, homoeopathy calls it the law of similars.

Homoeopathy has other principles like the minimum dose, the infinitesimal dose, totality of symptoms, Hering's law of cure, etc. But every one of these rests on the soundness of the law of similars. Without the law of similars there is no homoeopathy. But it would be a mistake to just look at this law from the perspective of what can create an illness can also cure it, for this is selling the law short. Likes not only *cure* likes, they also attract likes. Why? Because the cure exists in the similimum.

A problem that is unrecognised is a problem that cannot be fixed. If we have some part of our nature that needs to be addressed and overcome, the only way of recognising its existence is to have it forced in our face at a level that cannot be ignored; that is what we call a problem. This problem will have the same character as the miasm that is in us. A problem is the externalisation of the miasmatic pattern that surrounds us. A suspicious person who drives their partner crazy with their questioning begins to lose the love and respect they once had because their partner feels mistrusted and controlled, the self-fulfilling prophecy. In the Hawaiian shamanic system called Huna, they declare that, "energy flows where attention goes".

Everyone has a distinct miasmatic energy around them and this energy governs much of our personality. That means that much of our character is merely the miasm at work. This can be seen by predictable problems and generic thought patterns by different patients from the same miasmatic group. At first I found this lack of individuality disturbing. I was raised on the philosophy that every individual is like a clean slate, no words have been written on it, everything is yet to be formed, everything is in the process of becoming but nothing has been determined. There is comfort in this philosophy: it means everything about you, your outlook, your temperament, whether you are a happy person or not, a fatalist or an optimist, all this and more will be formed throughout the course of your life by the random events and circumstances that happen to you. No wonder so much emphasis is placed on education, stimulation and upbringing. Every one of us has the potential to become successful, learned, well paid leaders if we want it badly enough. This view is not unlike the Freudian concept where our personalities become the sum of all the collective domestic dramas that occurred through our formative years.

Both philosophies share the belief that events dictate personality. These theories have been readily adopted as they serve a useful purpose. Like the Pasteurian "germ theory" they are empowering, though it is true that Pasteur's theory only really empowers the medical profession. The "clean slate" empowers every individual as it places the future into the hands of the individual. Historically this is significant because after centuries of feudalism and class oppression the average person finally had a philosophy that didn't run them down or predetermine their future. The only problem with the theory is that it is wrong.

The miasms show that people are anything but "clean slates". Every one of us at the moment of conception receives massive amounts of information, every possibility is catered for before we take our first breath, within the embryo, the old man already exists. It is a fallacy to assume that life circumstances alone turned a happy child into a depressed adult, without acknowledging an inherent potential towards depression. Was there ever a stage, from the embryo onwards, when a Down's syndrome child was not Down's syndrome? At no stage in our life from first breath to last can we ever extend beyond our potential. There was a case recently where a little girl suffered a "breakdown" after viewing a horror movie. Of course many were up in arms about the nature of the movie itself and cries of tougher censorship were called for. I am not saying the movie was blameless but it can only trigger something that already exists.

I don't believe the miasms determine our future in a fatalistic way, but they most certainly determine our instinctive response to stress. Not only do I think that effects of stress are miasmatically determined but so are the causes of the stress. To clarify by example, syphilis has around it an element of violence. This does not mean they are violent people, as an aura or energy is not necessarily a literal thing, but violence in any of its forms has the potential to follow the syphilitic around. This aura or energy in relation to the miasms is referred to in this book as a miasmatic theme, an energy that encircles and saturates the person. For example, if two people, were walking down the street, one psoric the other syphilitic and a mugger was lurking, the syphilitic person would most likely be the one they would target. It must be stressed here that I am talking about statistical likelihoods *not* absolute certainties. Because a robbery or mugging is a violent act, the chance of the syphilitic, whose miasmatic theme contains violence, being the victim is significantly higher but certainly not exclusive.

Some people have things happen to them on a regular basis that are completely foreign to others. Some sit open-mouthed, completely awestruck at the continuous trend of bad luck experienced by others. This is a miasmatic theme. A series of events sewn together by a common thread that unless broken will recur over and over again.

You cannot run away from a miasmatic theme and it is almost impossible to eradicate. If we take our syphilitic patient as an example, she cannot decide to simply remove herself from the community in an effort to escape the violent segment of her miasm, for in each miasmatic theme there is a range of action and response. Violence may indeed belong to syphilis but so too does isolation.

The trends or themes that run throughout a miasm are varied, and more about this will be discussed, but it is important to address a few issues.

1. When discussing miasmatic themes we are not talking about certainties.

2. Miasmatic themes are *not* prophesies.

3. Miasmatic themes are varied and the ways they can be exhibited innumerable.

4. Miasmatic themes are issues not caricatures

Miasms offer the practitioner a valuable insight into their patient's lives and help clarify why certain events and misfortunes occur. So integrated into us have the miasms become that discovering the dividing line between the miasm and true nature is almost impossible, but Hahnemann has left with us a legacy that transcends even his expectations. Thanks to homoeopathy we have a chance at being able to decipher the real from the illusion.

I would like to take a quote from *The Tibetan Book of Living and Dying* Of course there is no reference to the miasms per se but here the term ego could easily mean the same as miasm.

Two people have been living in you all your life. One is the ego, garrulous, demanding, hysterical, calculating; the other is the hidden spiritual being, whose still voice of wisdom you have only rarely heard or attended to... As the voice of your discriminating awareness grows stronger and clearer, you will start to distinguish between its truth, and the various deceptions of the ego... more and more, then, instead of the harsh and fragmented gossip that has been talking to you all your life, you will find yourself hearing in your mind the clear directions of the teachings, which inspire, admonish, guide and direct you at every turn... A new life utterly different from that when you were masquerading as your ego begins in you... When your amnesia over your identity begins to be cured, you will realise finally that dak dzin, grasping at self, is the root cause of all your suffering.

The miasm, like the ego, is a trickster. Because the miasm is in our genes we identify with it and believe that we and it are one and the same, but this is a mistake, in fact nothing could be further from the truth. The very fact that I am able to talk about miasmatic themes at all is because there is a noticeable predictability about them. Each miasm has similar likes and dislikes, people will tell you about their drives and motivations not realising that these are common to many others from their miasmatic group. Even the type of words a patient may choose to describe their life can become hauntingly familiar. These things have commonalities to them, even though we may think they are us, this thinking is false. Hahnemann wrote the most important things in a case are the rare, strange and peculiar, as they are the symptoms that tell us about the patient rather than the disease, and the same process is in motion here. We need to find out what is common to the miasm in order to see what is truly individual within each person. Homoeopaths have always been wise enough not to fall into the trap of donating all one's time and energy to the study of common pathological symptoms as they tell you nothing but the bare minimum about the sufferer. Why should the miasms, the basis of all illness, follow different rules to every other malady? These are the rules of nature and as such are set and incontrovertible whether acute, chronic or in this case genetic.

People talk in language common to their miasm. People have dreams common to their miasm. They have taste buds common to their miasm. They have facial features common to their miasm. People have hobbies, interests, musical tastes, sexual preferences, aspirations and goals, common to their miasm. But a miasm is a disease and should always be treated as such. We know it's a disease because it does what all diseases do, it destroys individual character. Alzheimer's disease ravages the individual until there is nothing left but senility. Some diseases replace life with pain; others will substitute an old well-known personality with another nowhere near as pleasant. Disease can make people bitter, helpless or lonely. Some diseases destroy while others torment. There are no good diseases, and there are no good miasms. A disease and/or a miasm share one goal; to take away vitality and to use your energy for its own selfish growth, just like a virus. All diseases inhibit and erode growth, freedom and individuality. All diseases stem from the chronic miasms, so at its most fundamental level it would be true to say there are only seven real diseases in existence, each one of them a miasm. All the multitude of pathologies that fill the medical libraries are merely expressions of the miasms. All diseases, irrespective of name and title, belong to a miasmatic group.

Consider the following quote by Kent:

A patient of twenty-five years of age, with gravest inheritances, with twenty pages of symptoms, and with only symptoms to furnish an image of sickness, is perfectly curable if treated in time. After being treated there will be no pathological results; he will go on to old age without any tissue destruction. But that patient if not cured at that early age will take on disease results in accordance with the circumstances of this life and his inheritances. If he is a chimney sweep he will be subject to the disease peculiar to chimney sweeps. If she is a housemaid she will be subject to the disease peculiar to housemaids, etc. That patient has the same disease he had when he was born. This array of symptoms represents the same state before the pathological conditions have been formed as after. And it is true, if he has liver disease or brain disease or any of the many tissue changes that they call disease, you must go back and procure these very symptoms before you can make a prescription. Prescribing for the results of disease causes changes in the results of disease, but not in sickness except to hurry its progress...We will see peculiarities running through families. In the beginning is this primary state which is presented only by signs and symptoms, and the whole family needs the same remedy or a cognate of that remedy; but in one member of the family the condition runs to cancer, in another to phthisis, etc., but all from the same common foundation. This fundamental condition which underlies the diseases of the human race must be understood.

According to Kent a miasm exists long before any pathological result develops. A miasm is the predisposition to get sick as well as the direction that the sickness takes; he has no real regard for the name of the disease and even less for simple organic explanations regarding its origin. As can be seen from the above quotes, to Kent the miasms are inherited tendencies toward disease development.

Notice that Kent mentions in the last quoted paragraph two potentially fatal chronic diseases originating from the same familial or miasmatic weakness. The disease classification or term, whether it be acute or chronic, is only relevant to a certain degree. When a disease like cancer occurs in a family we must not automatically assume that the cancer miasm is dominant, for in Kent's example another member of that same family also acquired tuberculosis. The main trend is one of destruction and that is what a miasmatic prescriber would focus on.

As the internal is so is the external, and the external cannot be except as the result of the internal...The internal state of man is prior to that which surrounds him; therefore, environment is not cause; it is only, as it were, a sounding board; it only reacts upon and reflects the internal... Things flow in the direction he wants them to flow... The image of his own interior self comes out in disease.

- Kent

CHAPTER 3

Homoeopathic Genetics Miasmatic Inheritance

Just as when the ground luminosity dawned at the moment of death, here too in the bardo of dharmata, liberation cannot be taken for granted. For when the brilliant light of wisdom shines out, it is accompanied by a display of simple, comforting, cosy sounds and lights, less challenging and overwhelming than the light of wisdom. These dim lights – smoky, yellow, green, blue, red, and white – are our habitual, unconscious tendencies accumulated by anger, greed, ignorance, jealousy and pride. These are the emotions that create the six realms of ... The cosy lights, the invitation of our habitual tendencies, lure us toward a rebirth, determined by the particular negative emotion that dominates our karma and our mindstream.

- The Tibetan Book of Living and Dying

This quote from *The Tibetan Book of Living and Dying* more than any other passage outside of homoeopathic literature highlights the true essence of exactly what a miasm is. All miasms, not just psora, are grooves and faults. They are the imperfections that influence and modify potential, they dictate life events and direct their consequences.

In the opening quote, when a person dies, the soul leaves its body behind and spends a certain amount of time by itself. This isolation can be confusing and confronting. Soon some colours or sounds begin to emerge. These colours and sounds are manifestations of emotion, visible or audible representations of the negative instinctual passions that have tortured us for lifetimes. Unrecognised in regards to their emotional association, these tones or colours feel comforting, seductive and strangely familiar. Drawn towards the colour or tone we resonate with the most, we suddenly find ourselves ensnared into yet another rebirth, again burdened by the stigma of this negative emotion we are seemingly unable to overcome. If we had transcended our individual instinctive tendencies all the colours and all the tones would be unappealing, they would not beckon us and we would be free to move on.

Understanding this concept of rebirth via an emotional manifestation into colour, allows us to appreciate what is termed "karmic vision".

How is it that we come to be alive as human beings? All beings who have similar karma will have a common vision of the world around them ... Each one of us is a complex summation of habits and past actions, and so we cannot but see things in our own uniquely personal way. Human beings look much the same but perceive things utterly differently, and we each live in our own unique and individual worlds.

This statement has such resonance and profundity to our homoeopathic purpose that if the language was changed into homoeopathic terms it would be one of the best descriptions of the homoeopathic constitution yet written.

"All beings who have a similar karma will have a common vision of the world around them..." this is a perfect and precise description of what is meant by a miasmatic theme. A miasmatic theme is a common idea, fear or desire shared by those who have a similar karma, or in homoeopathic terms belong to the same miasmatic group. Hence there will be themes or trends, as themes can also be physicals, which most people who belong to a miasm will share.

Another way of comprehending the ramifications and impact of a miasm is by understanding that everything that is ever done within a person's lifetime, everything they ever see and everything they ever hear will be influenced by the miasm that interprets it. If a person is psoric, then everything will have a psoric accent. This means that while it can never be said that only psorics will do this or all sycotics will do that, it is true to state that even though a psoric and a sycotic person may team up to accomplish the same thing, how they accomplish the task, what they expect to gain from it as well as what motivated them to take it on in the first place will be entirely different. Miasmatic understanding is not about outcomes, it is about understanding motivations.

A miasmatic theme is our version of karmic vision. Once rebirth occurs a person who has been drawn into the green spectrum, for example, will return with the same old instinctual tendencies that all greens suffer from. This pattern is desperately hard to break as it involves seeing yourself and the world through different eyes from the ones you've been given in order to have any hope at all of liberation. A green sees the world and everyone in it, each and every event that occurs, through green and only green eyes. Each individual may see the same event, but how it is interpreted will be entirely different.

Interpretations are based entirely on previous experience. One can only make an evaluation by reference to the past. Imagine trying to explain to someone that you have just seen a life form from outer space, but this life form has no similarity to anything that has ever existed on earth, it is completely unique, indeed even its colour is a colour that you have never seen. It has no odour and it made a sound that could not be imitated. How can you explain what you have seen without a previous comparison to equate it to? Everything that is ever seen or done is always matched and reviewed against previous experience. A new experience must have some similarity to a past event otherwise it will disorient the senses. Most new experiences have only a slight variation from the ones of the past so the event can be accepted. This is how a body of knowledge is built; it takes time to gain experience and experience to gain wisdom.

What if someone's past experience is entirely different from your own? If their memories and truths are completely different? Obviously their world as well as what exists in it will be different from the world you inhabit. Let's take it a little further; what happens if beliefs gained through experience are inherited? If acquired knowledge from previous generations is handed down genetically rather than buried with the corpse? After all, every other facet of our makeup is transferred and stored genetically, why would knowledge, the most important survival tool of all, be the only exception? That would mean that the way any individual will view the world and how they interact with it, together with the type of energy they will most likely emit were formed at the same time as the transference of every other piece of genetic material. Again this exemplifies why a person who is psoric is so from the moment of conception until the end of their time, but psora like all the miasms is a range of potential possibilities none of which is inevitable. Circumstance is the bridge between potential and development.

This may seem fatalistic at first but that would be a misconception. Free will survives and flourishes within this construct. The miasms inform us in advance of what the most likely consequences of our negative actions will be should we choose to continually succumb to them. Miasmatic themes are just words. Free will is their placement to form the story they will tell.

Miasmatic understanding shows that there is purpose in life, that life is not a series of random events or luck. It cannot explain everything of course, even homoeopathy has its limits, but it does provide as deep an understanding of human behaviour as any philosophy devised. Homoeopathy proves that there is a spiritual nature to mankind, how else can the infinitessimal dose work? To deny or shirk this understanding because it's embarrassing or because it conflicts with scientific medicine is to deny the truth. Homoeopathy shows that God is not a dirty word or an embarrassing one. Life does have meaning and events are not random.

As homoeopaths we understand that the cure is within the cause, not only in medicines but also in events. Only by recognising patterns do we finally ask ourselves "Why are these things happening?" It is not human nature to become self-reflective when everything is wonderful. Repeating events show us where and what to look for.

Why, then, cannot this vital force, efficiently affected through homoeopathic medicine, produce any true and lasting recovery in these chronic maladies even with the aid of the homoeopathic remedies which best cover their present symptoms; while this same force which is created for the restoration of our organism is nevertheless so indefatigably and successfully active in completing the recovery even in severe acute diseases? What is there to prevent this?

- Samuel Hahnemann

CHAPTER 4

The Various Ways Miasms are Clinically Applied

...there are presently two basic schools of thought in the homoeopathic profession regarding miasms: one which ignores the idea altogether, and another which accepts it thoughtlessly and therefore adopts a routine of prescribing in an attempt to "clear" the case of miasms.

- George Vithoulkas

The miasms are a construct, and like any other constructed theory, its design is to convey a message in a precise and easily recognisable way. One problem for homoeopaths is that the term miasm has a variety of different meanings. If I mention Hering's law, every homoeopath immediately knows what I am talking about; we are all speaking the same language. But this is not the case when it comes to the miasms as there are a number of ways they can be perceived and as such there needs to be some clarification of the different ways of understanding them. The following is a quick summary of the various ways miasmatic theory is currently applied.

1. MIASMATIC "CLEARING"

This practice entails the administration of an anti-miasmatic nosode. If a case is believed to be sycotic, then a prescription of Medorrhinum will be given at some stage in the case. In theory there is nothing wrong with this approach, however it is based on the notion that only a nosode actually touches the underlying miasm, as if for some reason the indicated constitutional remedy works on a different level or different area than a nosode. Hahnemann referred to many remedies as either anti-psoric or anti-sycotic, not just Psorinum or Medorrhinum. If nosodes alone are the only remedies capable of deep change, constitutional prescribing becomes worthless. Believing that the miasm is some different entity, divorced from what is causing a patient's symptoms, shows a complete misunderstanding of what disease is. Another form of this theory is to give a remedy to "clear" or 'wipe out' a miasm. Medorrhinum is administered to "get rid" of the sycotic layer so the constitutional medicine can do its work. But the miasm is *causing* all the symptoms, so if the miasm were truly able to be eradicated – which would be fantastic – there would be nothing to prescribe for. The miasm **is the disease**, you do not remove it to get a clearer picture of the case.

All chronic illness has its origin in the miasms, that's the major message of the last edition of the *Organon*. If a miasm could be removed, which it cannot, but let's for the sake of argument pretend, then all any person on the earth would need for the total eradication of all suffering and disease, is to take one dose of Medorrhinum, Syphilinum, Tuberculinum, Psorinum and

Carcinosin. That would eradicate the cause of all illness as the miasms are now removed, but experience denies this theory; life shows that miasms can be tempered, but no one has ever been permanently freed from their grip. They cannot be "cleared".

2. THE LAYERS APPROACH

This method is the most widespread and commonly used in homoeopathy. In essence the layers approach springs from statements Hahnemann made regarding the treatment of chronic illness in both the *Organon* and in *Chronic Diseases*. Hahnemann talks of treating "complex" cases with anti-psoric medicines firstly then moving on to the relevant anti-syphilitic or anti-sycotic remedies, as the case requires. He saw each miasm as a separate entity and as a consequence treated them independently from each other. The layers theory implies that every individual has every miasm in them. Each effective remedy will remove the one layer which that remedy resonates with, which is then replaced by the next underlying miasm. This philosophy is the basis behind the breaking up of cases into their parts for minute miasmatic assessment. In this way a person may present with a tumour (cancer) which is producing bone pain (syphilis) night sweats (tubercular) and a skin rash (psora). The inadequacy of this method rests in the fact that it is a continuum that has no conclusion.

3. ACQUIRED MIASMATIC DISEASE

This version of the miasms is a kind of 'never been well since' adaptation. It is designed to suit those cases where an actual infection with a malady deemed miasmatic has occurred. For example, if a patient has been diagnosed with tuberculosis then Tuberculinum is administered, if they have had gonorrhoea, then a dose of Medorrhinum is given. Kent warns about this indiscriminate use of nosodes based on this premise as he believes this method's theoretical basis is both fallacious and simplistic.

4. FAMILY HISTORY OF AN ACQUIRED MIASMATIC DISEASE

This is an extension of the personally acquired miasmatic disease theory but perhaps more reliable as it can display a trend. Based on the same assumptions, this method is applied when a patient's family history contains a disease like cancer or tuberculosis. As will be shown, a history of cancer in the family does not necessarily mean that you or your patient belong to that same miasm. But it is true to say that a strong ancestral history of cancer, especially if it is on *both* sides of the family, is enough to alert the practitioner to the possibility that their patient may belong to this miasmatic group. This shows the importance of an extended repertoire of chronic diseases based on modern-day pathology. We know that the cancer miasm, for example, strongly, but never solely, influences the development of diabetes or chronic fatigue. All the miasms need a pool of modern pathology such as this to provide another possible miasmatic indicator, as long as it is always remembered as a guide and never taken as a certainty.

5. MISMANAGED OR SUPPRESSED DISEASE

Another popular opinion regarding the nature of miasms is the view that a miasm is any disease that has been driven back into the system by medical mismanagement and suppression. This opinion stems directly from Hahnemann. Throughout the fifth and sixth editions of the *Organon* as well as in his *Chronic Diseases*, Hahnemann highlights how many diseases have been made far more dangerous because of ignorant and hazardous treatment. Hahnemann accuses medicine of continually disallowing nature to throw symptoms on to the surface of the skin where they can do the least harm by treatments that serve to drive the illness into the internal economy where it can wreak havoc. The disease then occupies the whole internal nature of the sufferer and becomes engrafted to their vital force. From here, the disease can influence the next generation as its spirit is passed on with inheritance. This position on the miasms gives rise to the proposal that new miasms are being created every day. Hence there is an AIDS miasm and a cortisone miasm and an asthma miasm and so on. In this representation any drug or disease can, if mismanaged or engrafted through continuance, become a miasm.

6. ALPHA AND OMEGA

There exists a hypothesis that when confronted with a case that is thoroughly confusing, either because a patient's symptoms are all over the place or because there are no real or clear symptoms, the administration of a nosode will help arrange the symptoms into a more discernible pattern, or will bring to life a tired and expressionless case by throwing symptoms out on to the surface where they can be observed. Likewise there also exists the idea that after the successful completion of a case the closing prescription should be the relevant nosode to theoretically limit the impact coming from the underlying miasm.

7. THE MIASMS AS A STATE OF STRESS REACTION

This is a more modern approach used by some homoeopaths. Here a miasm is interpreted as a stage of response, like the predictable stages of response to crisis, such as anger, denial and acceptance. The miasms in this model represent a stage in which a patient finds themselves stuck, unable to move through the process until the appropriate medicine is given. This emotional response now becomes the only way this patient can respond to stress, regardless of its cause. As an example Rajan Sankaran writes:

This response therefore is the best indicator of the miasm. I also call this response the "coping mechanism" and this is best seen in relation to the chief complaint as the patient's attitude toward the illness. If his attitude is one of panic, the miasm in the case is likely to be acute. If it is hopeful, it is likely to be psora. If he adopts an attitude of resigned acceptance, avoidance or cover up it may be sycosis and if he feels hopeless and destructive it may be syphilis. This miasm can then be confirmed throughout the rest of the case as an action taken in response to the depth of the sensation perceived.

8. THE SINGLE DOMINANT MIASM

This theory presents the hypothesis that each individual is primarily influenced by a single recognisable dominant miasm rather than a number or series of miasms all vying for control. This theory reasons that human beings have set guidelines and parameters to their behaviour. It tries to explain why each person will experience the same world differently as well as attempting to rationalise circumstance, behaviour and energy patterning.

But that the original malady sought for must be also of a miasmatic, chronic nature clearly appeared to me from this circumstance, that after it has once advanced and developed to a certain degree it can never be removed by the strength of any robust constitution, it can never be overcome by the most wholesome diet and order of life, nor will it die out of itself. But it is evermore aggravated, from year to year, through a transition into other and more serious symptoms, even till the end of man's life.

- Samuel Hahnemann

CHAPTER 5

The Single Dominant Miasm Theory

As cure commonly means the removal of some evil, distress or disability, its scope is broad and its attainment idealistic. What seems so sure a cure today we may tomorrow know as a recovery only, for it is one thing to hold the vital forces well in hand, but quite another to eradicate disease. While cleanliness has done much to limit new accretions to psora, syphilis and sycosis, it has accomplished nothing toward removing the death stamp which these miasms have fixed upon the human cell for thousands of generations; nor will it. Only a similarly acting, non-self-propagating substance can stimulate the cell to throw off these poisons which have fastened themselves upon it and which daily ripen a rich harvest for the surgeon and the undertaker.

- Cyrus M Boger

This chapter discusses the theory of a single dominant miasm. This notion may be the most controversial claim of the book because it conflicts with the layers theory of the miasms which is the most accepted of all the various theories.

The layers approach, although more accepted, fails to offer any real solution to the problems faced by homoeopaths every day in their clinic, and unless miasmatic philosophy manifests as practical action, no real clinical purpose is served and it remains a topic rather than a tool. The layers approach attempts to understand the miasms in a case. It highlights the key symptoms of the case and matches each symptom individually to its supposedly indicated miasm. For example, "This patient suffers from depression (syphilis) but they also have fixed ideas (sycosis) and like to travel (tubercular)", but in reality, how useful is it to know this? Especially when nine times out of ten, the remedy is chosen according to the symptom totality without any reference to which miasm it belongs to anyway. This miasmatic prelude to remedy selection amounts to nothing but a waste of time. It serves no practical value to go through a case bit by bit in order to break down each pathological component into its corresponding miasm. A constitutional remedy is never selected simply because it contains a lot of particulars. The nature of the patient, their mental and general features are always the overriding qualities, far outweighing any particulars or named pathology present in the case. Why should the rules be changed in relation to the miasms?

One of the ways history has solved this conundrum has been to adopt a theory that states that every person and every remedy has every miasm in it. Therefore Sulphur is a suitable remedy for cases of psora and sycosis and syphilis, because if you look closely enough at Sulphur as a remedy you will see bits of all of these miasms. The same can be said for Thuja, Mercury, Lycopodium and Arsenicum, etc. What is the point of classification if the end result is so broad you learn nothing from it? This is the same as classifying everything that is organic but does not move as a plant and everything that does as an animal. This classification process sheds no light as to the type of plant or animal, its habits and so on. Everything may as well be put under the even broader classification of "stuff". Whilst this sounds ridiculous, it is no less ridiculous than saying that all people have all miasms as do all remedies so it's important to get the right one!

I once attended a lecture on the topic of clarifying the miasms. This same common but misleading layers model was the central focus. It was defined quite erroneously as 'the only miasmatic model in use'. The same complex approach was adopted, breaking down each symptom piece by piece. Soon the class white board looked like a massive spider web with lines linking each symptom to its miasm. And in the end, by the lecturer's own admission, the remedy was selected on the basis of the presenting symptom picture. This can be done without any miasmatic understanding at all.

The miasms serve no real function if their influence is not catered for. It is for precisely this reason that Hering and countless others since have said either openly or in their own minds, "What does it matter whether the miasms are catered for or not provided I select the right rubrics and prescribe the correct medicine.

If practitioners are happy with the layers model and find it aids them in their remedy selection then I encourage them to continue with it, but I was at the point where the existence of miasms was more confusing than helpful. Either I was going to stop thinking about the miasms altogether, or a more plausible and easily understood approach had to be adopted and it must serve a practical purpose.

At its most basic level, the hypothesis underpinning this whole system is the proposition of a single dominant miasm.

This means each individual may have a number of symptoms from a number of miasms, but one of those miasms will be in a dominating position and as a consequence it is that particular miasm which the remedy will need to cater for.

The dominant miasm is the miasm with the most influence; it asserts its authority over all others. There can only ever be one dominant miasm in the one body at the one time; the laws of homoeopathy tell us so.

1. *If the two dissimilar diseases meeting together in the human being be of equal strength, or still more if the older one be the stronger, the new disease will be repelled by the old one from the body and not allowed to affect it.*

2   *Two diseases similar to each other [Two Similar Diseases in the Sixth Edition] can neither (as is asserted of dissimilar disease in I) repel one another, nor (as has been shown of dissimilar disease in II) suspend one another, so that the old one shall return after the new one has run its course; and just as little can two similar diseases (as has been demonstrated in III respecting dissimilar affections) exist beside each other in the same organism, or together form a double complex disease.*

Every one of us has character traits that are common to others. Often these will take the form of likes or dislikes, hobbies, fears or phobias, perhaps even an entire belief system. Not a single mannerism do we have that is ours and ours alone, there is always someone else who will share some aspect of our character. But while another individual may share one or two of our personal mannerisms, that same individual will not share all of them nor will the ones they do share be in exactly the same proportion. When it comes to the miasms the subtleties are precisely the same. They all share certain pathologies and they all seem to have some characteristics in common although many of these of course belong to the human condition. Each individual miasmatic family has its own unique and independent character traits that may be mimicked by another miasm but its exact identity can never be precisely replicated.

An individual's basic nature and character remain relatively constant throughout life. Events and circumstances occur throughout one's lifetime that will serve as moderators to behaviour; we learn what we can get away with, who we can trust and who we cannot, we become smarter at satisfying our needs, but by and large our essence remains the same. This means there is an element of stability in character, we are at all times exactly who we are, we are never approximately who we are even when complying with others or putting on an act.

Each miasm has some unique behavioural qualities, for example sycosis contains a strong element of suspicion and jealousy, but for these emotions to be regarded as a miasmatic theme they must be continuous and unjustified. Jealousy or suspicion is an appropriate and natural response to certain conditions, but a jealous reaction does not necessarily mean a jealous person, hence to take away the cause is to take away the reaction. A miasmatic theme by contrast is when a person continually exhibits the response without the cause being present. This is the difference between being jealous and being a jealous person. A jealous person will bring this feeling into every relationship they have. A person who is jealous by nature, or suspicious, placid, depressed or optimistic, usually stays so for most of their lives.

Facial features also develop early and like character stay relatively stable throughout life. Appearance is genetically determined and as such is heavily influenced like all things by the miasm. If syphilis can alter bone structure for generations to come, it must influence our DNA. But why should syphilis be the only miasm to do this? Syphilis is no stronger than any of the other miasms. All the miasms become part of our DNA, which is why we are influenced by them on all levels of existence. For a person to continually change their miasm would mean that they are continually changing their genetic material and that isn't possible.

To highlight how the miasms could not possibly be in a state of constant flux and change I would like to refer to genetic illness. If a child is born mentally retarded it would be fair to suggest that the syphilitic miasm is showing a prevailing presence. But if everyone truly has all the miasms in them, and they are constantly revolving in an ebb and flow continuum, then we should expect a mentally retarded person to go through both psoric and sycotic phases, not to continually exhibit the syphilitic only.

But in practice this phenomenon never occurs. Never at any stage in this person's life will the syphilitic miasm loosen its grip and free them, even momentarily, from their retardation. Syphilis will always be dictating the genetic terms. This person was born with a syphilitically dominant miasm and they will end their life exactly the same way. Nature is full of genetically inherited diseases and not one of them will fluctuate in and out of being, they are immovable and absolute. The genetic disease does not change because the single dominant miasm responsible for it does not change.

Homoeopathic literature has numerous cases where successful treatment has changed a patient's whole personality, but what is really meant by this? Are we suggesting that in both personality and appearance this patient bears no resemblance to the person they used to be? Or are we using it as a way of highlighting how positive and energetic this same patient has become? If a miasm influences appearance, then a patient's appearance would change in accordance to each miasmatic layer lifted, but this does not happen.

Homoeopathy is all about balance, this is what our remedies do; they do not change intrinsic character, they modify it. No homoeopathic remedy, no matter how well selected, has the ability to change who we are, but it can certainly help make us the best we can be.

Genetic inheritance and the miasms are interchangeable versions of one another. The study of the miasms is the study of homoeopathic genetics. But homoeopathic genetics is not the same as its allopathic counterpart; homoeopathic genetics is the study of psychological and biological trends.

A person's dominant miasm does not change after the administration of the correct remedy, but the influence of that miasm is certainly lessened. Everyone has traits that do not work in their best interests. Examples of such traits might be a tendency to withhold emotion or to form addictions. The right remedy can help overcome these tendencies, and with knowledge and willpower an extended state of quiescence can exist. But these traits will always exist even if subdued, an alcoholic is an alcoholic even when not drinking because the tendency is the disease and the miasm creates the tendency. A tendency is never eradicated, it is subdued, and this is what a remedy does. To highlight, very few people are ever only addicted to one thing, if one outlet of addiction is taken away another will replace it, the real disease is the addictive tendency.

The single dominant miasm remains constant, miasms *do not* swap and change. A person who is syphilitic is so from birth to death, if it were otherwise we would see all the other miasms and their flow-on effects – emotional, mental, pathological and appearance–go through waves of change every few months or years. This does not occur because miasmatic rotation is a fallacy and the sooner it is dropped as a concept the more organised homoeopathy will become.

As the name suggests the single dominant miasm theory means only one miasm holds an influence, hence the characteristics and symptoms belonging to that particular miasm will be the majority of symptoms your patient will present with. Their problems and difficulties will be coming from the influence of their dominant miasm. Nobody can belong to two different miasmatic groups at the same time, you cannot be psoric and sycotic. You can, however, be syco-psoric, but as will be discussed, this miasm is an entity in its own right. A complex miasm is regarded as a single miasm and as such has become the single dominant influencing miasm.

The single dominant miasm theory is also important because it means patients and remedies can be classified into distinct, recognisable and unchanging groups. This introduces an element of certainty that was lacking before its development. For example, after a repertorisation has been completed there will often be six or seven remedies vying for contention. Imagine these remedies include Sulphur, Silica, Pulsatilla, Tuberculinum, Arsenicum and Phosphorus. With miasmatic prescribing each one of the above remedies belongs to and represents a particular miasm group. Let's pretend our make-believe patient belongs to the cancer miasm. According to the above repertorisation there are only two remedies, not six to consider. If cancer is the dominant miasm, and this will be decided by the facial features, then Silica and Arsenicum are the only two remedies we need look at. None of the other remedies, no matter how seemingly well indicated, will touch the underlying miasm driving the case, only a well-selected remedy, in accordance with the symptoms and the underlying miasm, can do this. Of course this does not mean that a well-selected non-miasmatic remedy will do nothing, after all it still matches the presenting symptoms, but there is a real difference between removing symptoms and restoring health.

As students we read accounts of how the well-indicated remedy failed to relieve. But how can this be so? These practitioners matched all the presenting symptoms of the case to the remedy and yet it still failed. Misunderstanding miasmatic knowledge is the main reason this occurs.

There are some crucial facts to understanding disease.

1. Chronic disease is always constitutional. A constitutional remedy is the combination of life circumstance and the inherited miasm

2. Miasmatic illness is the only real disease as it lies at the foundation of constitutional prescribing; it is the sum total of all inherited strengths and weaknesses.

This being the case, how can a prescription be regarded as accurate if the miasm is not being catered for? The underlying miasm must be addressed, otherwise "well-selected" remedies will not be a true similimum and oftentimes will fail. Prescribing a constitutional medicine indicated on both symptom totality and underlying miasm guarantees deeper results than symptom prescribing alone.

CHAPTER 6

Pathology and the Miasms

The suffering that frightens and terrifies man, detracting from him in various ways, and which we call "sickness", is manifested in each individual by his own personal characteristics, but if observed closely and carefully in humanity as a whole, is seen to yield determinate patterns. These special ways of "being sick" compel us to formulate groupings with a common constitutional basis which is manifested in these groups of individuals through similar pathological expressions.

- Dr P S Ortega

The three miasms are essentially just descriptors for the three major avenues of physiological response, just as the inflammatory response is a predictable non-changing reaction to physical trauma. When the body is thrown out of order there are only a limited number of ways it can react. These reactions include: hypo-function, hyper-function and dysfunction, or placed another way they are; too little, too much, destructive or inappropriate. When viewed in this way it can be seen that nearly all pathologies are an example of one, or a combination, of these responses. Hahnemann's miasmatic model is another way of applying specific professional jargon to these three reactions.

Syphilis was the first of the miasms described by Hahnemann for the reason that its effect above all others was the most obvious. As described in earlier chapters, it was syphilis that left its indelible imprint on the next generation for all to see. It was syphilis that so obviously maimed both physically and mentally its victims not only by contagion but also by heredity. Psora on the other hand had to be arrived at through an intellectual process of elimination.

Because psora is hypo-functional or "lack of" its presence is not obvious unless you know quite specifically what you are looking for. To many authors, Roberts included, psora doesn't have any real pathology. Some have even taken this further to suggest that psora is essentially the fear of disease but once a pathology actually manifests, another miasm must be responsible to bring it to structural life as psora is defined as being functional disturbance only. How this philosophy took shape is a little uncertain, suffice to say it does not coincide with what Hahnemann believed psora to be. Hahnemann thought psora to be a hydra-headed monster capable of all sorts of human atrocities and disfigurations. Hahnemann believed psora to be the greatest enemy known to man and the cause of innumerable amounts of suffering.

So which is accurate? Does psora cause pathological change or doesn't it? The answer lies in the remedies that epitomise the psoric miasm best. Let's take Sulphur for example, the well known "prince of the anti-psorics". According to *Phatak's Materia Medica* Sulphur includes pathological outcomes such as cancer of the breast or uterus, asthma, pleurisy, pneumonia, pericarditis, hydrocele and ulcers together with some mental pathologies or states such as, delusions of grandeur, depression and suicidal tendencies, all from a remedy that is meant to exemplify a miasm that has no physical power. Obviously the acceptance of the notion that psora is functional only is misguided and contains a line of thought that would only serve to confuse miasmatic understanding rather than clarify it.

Likewise Lycopodium, another great anti-psoric, sometimes called the vegetable Sulphur, contains within its sphere of influence pathological conditions and states such as paralysis, cancer, emaciation, meningitis and stomach ulcers. Even Psorinum itself, the ultimate representative of the miasm contains pathological conditions which include ulcers, boils, cancer and gout; even spina bifida can be a product of psora.

With the layers approach to the miasms, cancer or any ulcerations are considered to be the syphilitic phase of illness, but as the psoric remedies themselves show, they are capable of far more that just 'wrong or incorrect thoughts'. Psora has more than enough power to create actual disease.

A commonly asked question concerning matters of miasmatic pathology is, "Wouldn't spina bifida be an example of the syphilitic influence of the remedy?" The short answers to this is no. Because a remedy has some degeneration within its extent of possibility does not make it a syphilitic remedy. It is simply not true that all remedies contain syphilis and sycosis within them, nor do all people. Remedies are agents that are needed to restore balance when a stress has become too powerful for our defences to keep in check and harmony cannot be restored by our own power or ability alone. The pathology that has arisen out of these circumstances will always be in direct proportion and reflect the event itself. A strong and prolonged stress must produce a reaction in direct proportion to it. It is inconceivable to assume that somebody who is psoric will go through their entire life unscathed by events occurring around them simply because they are psoric. Are we to assume that nothing negative ever impacts upon psora? This is obviously not logical. Psora does react to circumstance; indeed many authors claim psora to be the most reactive of all the primary miasms, this is why it is the miasmatic impetus behind hay fever, allergies and the like. A miasm cannot be reactive and not reactive at the same time. The key is in understanding the force of the thrust needed to create the response. A healthy vital force should be able to evaluate and respond to an outside stress without having to answer it with strong physical signs and symptoms. Applying Hering's law, we understand that once physical signs and symptoms are produced the invading stress has already in some proportion overpowered the vital force, other strategic measures have been adopted in order to rid the body of the stress or invader.

The psoric vital force is strong, so therefore deep pathology and crippling signs and symptoms will be absent during the course of a normal, healthy, productive lifetime. However, should circumstances not be so favourable, psora is just as likely to develop signs and symptoms as any other miasm, but with such a strong vital force it is able to eject stress better than any other miasm. For deep pathology to occur, the impetus needs to be great*.

By contrast the syphilitic has an inherently weak or at least weaker constitution*. The syphilitic miasm like the psoric miasm can also create spina bifida, but the negative thrust needed in psora is infinitely greater due to the strength of its vital force than that needed to produce the same result in a syphilitic. Understanding this concept is vital to miasmatic prescribing, for without it we are back in a pathological paradigm that causes nothing but confusion. The presence of an actual condition or symptom does not automatically indicate the presence of the miasm that it may have traditionally been allocated to. The presence of a stomach ulcer does not mean that your patient is syphilitic. The presence of warts does not mean that either you or your patient is sycotic. The existence of eczema does not rule out every other miasm leaving only psora as the answer. No one single indicator alone can reveal the underlying miasm, only the

---

*Footnote 2008 - These conclusions were based on historically accepted concepts that psora is the least damaging miasm and syphilis the worst.

Clinical experience has not validated this assumption. The miasms have no hierarchical order. Psora and syphilis are both processes of defense no greater or lesser than each other or any other miasm.

---

sum total can determine this. And yet in seeming contrast to this, each one of the above can serve as an important indicator to their parent miasm when all other factors are included. Kent stated that pathology is the end result or ultimate in the disease process, but it must, by definition, bear a direct correspondence to the mental or miasmatic state that created it. Pathology, in order to be a guide to the miasm, must be taken into account but must never replace the generals of the case, no matter how dominant the pathology maybe.

A pathological name is no more a guide to the miasm than it is to a remedy; it can be used in the selection process but it should never form the basis of the selection. George Vithoulkas once stated that a person who develops leukaemia at a young age is more likely to have a complexity of miasms whereas a person who develops it at seventy is more likely to be psoric. This is an important statement which validates two important points just made.

1. Vithoulkas highlights that psora is not immune from disease, but psora's strong vital force means pathological development must have an overpowering co-factor such as age.

2. Disease names are not the same as miasmatic names. In this case cancer belonged to the psoric miasm, not the cancer miasm itself.

A cancer diagnosis does not mean the cancer miasm is dominant, in fact cancer as an illness belongs equally to all the miasmatic groups, including psora.

Before examining the miasmatic theme of psora, it is important at this point to explain an often overlooked detail. Students will sometimes state that the positive aspects of each miasm should be discussed. But miasms are diseases, and as such they do not possess any positive qualities. The miasms are inimical to life, they do not complement it nor do they add anything of value. Everything regarding the miasms is negative, there are no positive aspects*. This is a difficult concept to grasp because the miasms seem such a part of us that to deny them any worth seems to make ourselves worthless. It is true that some miasms have behavioural traits that are more socially acceptable, some are even expected or enforced, but this does not transform weights around our necks into wings on our backs. This becomes most confusing when dealing with psora, as a large part of their disposition is bright and sunny. I am not implying that this is a fault and agree that it is difficult to see why this trait should philosophically be regarded as a problem. There is no doubt that many miasmatic character traits can be rearranged to serve a useful purpose, and they can be channelled into areas where they will assist in a profitable manner, but this is using them, not transcending them.

*Footnote 2008 - Over six years has passed since writing this passage and I am now convinced that miasms are a system of defense rather than a disease or the result of a disease. The instinctive reaction to danger and stress that each miasm generates is not only beneficial but mandatory for survival.

Miasms when seen beyond the boundaries of disease display many positive traits which I have outlined in **Soul & Survival** (2008)

I also will choose their delusions, and I will bring their fears upon them; because when I called, none did answer; when I spake, they did not hear: but they did evil before mine eyes, and chose that in which I delighted not.

- Isaiah 66.4.

CHAPTER 7

The Number of Miasms

The three fundamental miasms of Hahnemann have been much derided,
but it is a great satisfaction to know that such things mostly come from
inexperienced or undeveloped minds. As year after year adds its share
of knowledge, conclusions change and the things disdained in youth
gradually become the frowning realities of maturer years. So it has
been and comes to be, that we look upon psora, syphilis and sycosis as
the poisonous fountain heads from which flow all our ills.

- Cyrus M Boger

One of the great practicalities of this miasmatic system
is to settle just how many miasms exist. This is
important because remedy classification into miasms cannot
be accomplished until a final decision regarding the number of
miasms has been reached. But this division cannot take place
until each miasmatic group becomes recognised and distinctive.
Its qualities should be discernible and separate, only then can
we notice a distinct difference between each miasmatic group
and why a remedy belongs to it. Until this takes place there is
no way of knowing which remedy belongs to which miasm,
so no comparative work can begin, and it is only through this
comparative detailing that a deep understanding of each
individual miasmatic family can be recognised.

Since their conception, miasms have played a pivotal role in homoeopathic philosophy but only a minor role in practical prescribing. This has always been the miasms' greatest weakness; an interesting theory but what do you do with it? Constantine Hering once wrote:

What important influence can it exert whether a homoeopath adopt the theoretical opinions of Hahnemann or not, so long as he holds the principal tools of the master and the Materia Medica of our schools? What influence can it have, whether a physician adopt or reject the psoric theory, so long as he always selects the most appropriate similar medicine possible?

JH Allen replies to this assertion:

The fact is, we cannot select the most similar remedy possible unless we understand the phenomena of the acting and basic miasms; for the true similia is always based upon the existing basic miasms, whether we be conscious or unconscious of the fact ... It is the difference between an intelligent warfare and fighting in the dark, it is no longer a battle in the mist.

The miasms according to some homoeopathic authors give clarification to a case, but the real question is what exactly do they clarify? It cannot be clearer identification of pathology, for even if we take a relatively minor condition like warts there are twelve remedies listed in **bold type** Some of these twelve remedies include Baryta.Carb, Calc, Merc.C and Sulphur. Even remedies like Aurum and Fluor Ac are listed in *italics*; not one of these remedies is commonly regarded as a purely sycotic medicine. The situation worsens if we extend into complicated pathologies. Miasms do not serve as great indicators in organic pathology, but they do help in identifying broad trends such as overgrowth or destruction. This being the case, their main area of illumination must lie elsewhere outside of pure pathology;

someone as astute as Hahnemann would never have committed so much time advocating and developing them if they were impractical.

Consider these words written by Hahnemann's own hand for they indicate more than just an interesting hypothesis:

I spent twelve years in investigating the source of this incredibly large number of chronic affections, in ascertaining and collecting certain proofs of this great truth ... before I had obtained this knowledge I could only teach how to treat the whole number of chronic diseases as isolated, individual maladies... so that every case of chronic disease was treated by my disciples according to the group of symptoms it presented ...How much greater cause is there now for rejoicing that the desired goal has been so much more nearly attained, inasmuch as the recently discovered and far more specific homoeopathic remedies for chronic affections arising from psora [properly termed antipsoric remedies ... and from among them the true physician can now select from his curative agents those whose medicinal symptoms correspond in the most similar [homoeopathic] manner to the chronic disease he has to cure; and thus, by the employment of [antipsoric] medicines more suitable for this miasm, he is enabled to render more essential service and almost invariably to effect perfect cure.

Hahnemann is specifically detailing a difference between symptom prescribing only, and prescribing for a patient based on the signs and symptoms of the case but also keeping the miasms as a focal point, formulating a prescription that specifically caters for both. Hahnemann claims quite categorically that if the miasms are not uppermost in the mind of the prescribing physician, the chances of affecting deep and lasting cure are reduced. Hahnemann is not saying that symptom diagnosis does not bring results, but what he and many other authors are saying, is that your success rate can be greatly improved by the inclusion of the miasms into your prescription.

Miasmatic understanding takes a prescription out of the "it looks a bit like" basket and gives each treatment a strong terra firma footing; by this I refer to the constitutional struggle each practitioner faces when a patient looks a "bit like" Arsenicum or a "bit like" Phosphorus. Miasmatic prescribing demands that each remedy must belong to the same miasmatic family as the patient you are treating. Hahnemann states that if you are dealing with a psoric case then a psoric remedy must be given, but it does not stop with psora, a sycotic patient must be given a sycotic medicine, a syphilitic patient, a syphilitic medicine, and so on, this is what similar similibus curantur is. Every homoeopath using the "symptom picture" method knows only too well how much any given case can look like a dozen or so different remedies even after a thorough repertorisation has taken place. Miasmatic understanding aids in remedy selection as it clarifies what medicine is appropriate for each individual case. Miasmatic diagnosis tells you that the remedy needed cannot possibly be x, y or z because your patient is sycotic and x, y and z are psoric.

I would like at this point to focus on the topic of miasmatic groups, and explain the number of miasms and the process used to reach a decision. The number of miasms in this model totals seven – hardly surprising considering this number's vibrational flavour. It is represented by the seven heavens, the amount of colours in the rainbow, seven chakras in the body, the number of notes on a musical scale and in a mandala; seven is the number of universal harmony.

In order to understand this next section three major points need to be acknowledged:

1. Hahnemann was accurate with his original miasmatic construct of psora, sycosis, and syphilis.

2. The addition of both the tubercular and cancer miasms is accurate and valid.

3. A finite number of miasmatic groups exists.

If each one of these points is acknowledged as legitimate then this miasmatic model is easily understood. Firstly let us look at Hahnemann's design of the three major miasms. Each one of these miasms is indisputable as all illness can be arranged into the areas of too little (psora), too much (sycosis) or dysfunctional and destructive (syphilis).

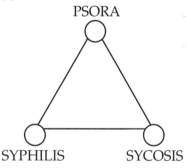

If we now include the addition of the tubercular miasm, the combinations of psora and syphilis, and place it in its appropriate position on the grid it looks like this:

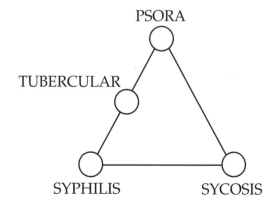

Next is the cancer or mixed miasm. This miasm is the combination of all of the three major miasms combined so we

have placed this miasmatic group in the middle of the drawing
to represent all of its influences.

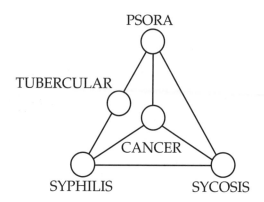

The foundation of this model rests entirely on Hahnemann's
deduction of the three primary miasms, this is then combined
with the Hahnemannian principle of "complex" diseases
as previously stated, and the remaining miasms manifest
themselves clearly.

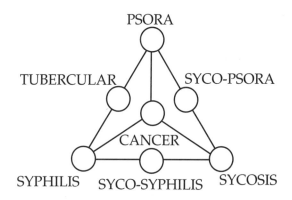

Expansion on the existing model could finally begin. With
a definite number of miasms settled upon, a stage had been
constructed in which the other miasms could now have their
properties and facial features identified and the table would be
complete.

This section of the project was in some ways the most difficult, as it became apparent that remedies renowned for their relevance to a particular miasm, did not belong to that particular group at all. In some instances this is understandable; in others a total rethink was required. When modern-day Homoeopaths refer to the very early works, it needs to be born in mind that Hahnemann believed that the majority of illnesses were of psoric origin. Indeed in *Chronic Diseases* Hahnemann writes the following to demonstrate this point:

The psora, which is now so easily and so rashly robbed of its ameliorating cutaneous symptom, the eruption of itch, which acts vicariously for the internal disease, has been producing within the last three hundred years more and more secondary symptoms, and indeed so many that at least seven-eighths of all the chronic maladies spring from it as their only source, while the remaining eighth springs from syphilis and sycosis ...

As a consequence of this statement, a disproportionate amount of remedies were allocated to the psoric miasm. After all, if seven-eighths of the population's symptoms are psoric, then seven-eighths of the remedies we use should also be psoric as should seven-eighths of the world's population. It is for reasons such as this that Hahnemann refers to nearly every medicine as an anti-psoric. But as brilliant as Hahnemann was, the miasms were still very much in their embryonic stage. Hahnemann attributed virtually everything to psora and this is part of the reason why so many homoeopaths at the time thought he had gone too far with this chronic disease business, hence Hering's remark as previously stated or one by Anthony Campbell where he writes in regards to the miasms theory: "A theory that tries to explain everything, explains nothing."

Too many problems combined with too many remedies invalidated the whole concept and left the miasm theory in an almost unworkable condition. Practitioners were divided and confused, some were loyal while others were openly hostile. Despite all this bickering and misunderstanding the chronic disease theory, like all things Hahnemann did, showed enlightened brilliance. The miasms were certainly in need of refining but they were also accurate and profound and offered great insight into the origins of disease.

CHAPTER 8

The Development of the New Miasms

Hahnemann first propounded this theory of disease to his closest colleagues, Dr Stapf and Dr Gross, in 1827, after having worked on it in private for some twelve years. The two men were horrified, fearing that such a wild idea would bring further contempt upon a homoeopathy already scoffed at because of the smallness of its doses. They pleaded with him not to publish it. However, for Hahnemann it had now become the bedrock of his medical theory: he could not suppress an explanation of disease which seemed to him to hold out the promise of a means to cure it. He published the ideas in Chronic Diseases in 1828, and shortly afterwards began to introduce into his practice methods of prescribing which were the consequence of the new theory.

Hahnemann's miasm theory, as it has become known, has been a difficulty for homoeopathic practitioners ever since. Some have responded like Stapf and Gross, with embarrassment; others have seen it as the most brilliant contribution to homoeopathy. Early English writers such as Dudgeon and Hughes were outright in their condemnation of it, while early Americans such as Allen and Kent seized upon it as the missing element in an otherwise perfect science. To this day many practitioners ignore it while others make it the foundation of their practice.

- Rima Handley

There exist seven miasms, five known and two unknown. With the five identified miasms there was an existing body of work from which information could be drawn, so further expansion into their themes and appearance was easier. There were already trade-mark symptoms and remedies that formed a foundation. If a patient responded exceptionally well at a constitutional level to remedies like Sulphur for instance it could immediately be suspected that the patient was psoric.

From this point a compilation of their looks and biography could be achieved and matched against other successful psoric cases to find common psoric ground. But when it came to either syco-psora and the syco-syphilis, no such precedence existed. Remedies had to be found that had an obvious combination of the two parent miasms in equal portions so a data base of information could be established.

To examine the syco-syphilitic miasm, two remedies that exemplified traits of both syphilis and sycosis were selected. A comparative examination could now be applied to find what features these remedies have in common. A repertorisation was later conducted on the common symptoms drawn from these remedies which enabled some new potentially additional syco-syphilitic remedies to arise. These in turn were assessed as to their suitability for categorisation into the syco-syphilitic group. The criteria for entry included having major generals found to be common within the syco-syphilitic group together with what was deemed to be characteristic mentals and essence or feel. This will be discussed in greater detail in coming chapters.

The two remedies selected as examples for the syco-syphilitic miasm were Lachesis and Staphisagria. The prime symptoms for deciding on Lachesis included their jealous and suspicious nature exemplifying sycosis combined with the septic and degenerative nature of syphilis. Staphisagria was selected because it also has an equal combination of sycosis and syphilis. Looking back on this humble beginning I am the first to recognise how naïve and inexperienced it seems, but it was a first step and, as luck or providence would have it, the choice was a valid one, as many successful clinical cases have proved the soundness of their syco-syphilitic allocation. Indeed these two remedies still present some of the best examples of this particular miasm.

From a comparison of these remedies, some interesting details were brought forth. In order to establish character, the major areas of examination referred to were the mentals and the generals. For example Morrison's *Desk Top Guide* lists under the generalities for Staphisagria: "General aggravation after taking a nap in the daytime, especially afternoon" and "General aggravation from sleep (irritable, unrefreshed, etc.)." Lachesis of course, from the same materia medica, has its tell tale "General aggravation during sleep or upon waking; sleeps into the aggravation." Staphisagria also has listed: "Masturbation". "Many sexual fantasies". "High sexual desire", "weak resistance", "sometimes promiscuous". While with Lachesis there is: "hyper-sexual", "nymphomania", "Masturbation", "excessive and precocious sexual development".

In Vermeulen, Staphisagria is expressed as: "sexually minded", "unsatisfied urge", "Intruding sexual thoughts; driving to masturbation". "Strong sexual fancies evening in bed; can only sleep after masturbation". "Often a history of sexual abuse". And with Lachesis he writes: "Strong sex drive, or high sexual standards [puritan, fanatic disapproval]". And "intense, passionate". "Goes to extremes".

As can be seen, a quite obvious sexual element presents

itself. A reference point had been formed, from here rubrics such as lasciviousness and generals such as worse after sleep could be repertorised, and the materia medica consulted. By this method a miasmatic flavour becomes noticeable. But repertorisation will only take you so far, and as all homoeopaths know, the real work is always done via the materia medica, for only the materia medica provides the understanding and character needed for this type of work. Thankfully syco-syphilis has a bold and easily recognisable essence, so establishing other remedies that belong to this miasmatic group was not overly difficult.

Whilst the syco-syphilitic miasm came together relatively easily, the same could not be said for the syco-psoric miasm. One of the main reasons for this is that narrowing down and defining psora is a deceptively difficult task. To simply refer to psora as a feigned philosopher that cannot fix their attention, prohibits the subtlety of character that modern-day homoeopaths need and depend upon. Perhaps these kinds of broad statements were all that were needed in earlier times, after all, psychological understanding was still in its infancy and most homoeopaths were doctors concerning themselves with diseases like scarlet fever, small pox and so on. However modern-day homoeopaths, particularly 'lay-practitioners' such as myself, rely on these intricacies of individuality to aid choices.

From previous work into the psoric miasm as well as a reasonably welldeveloped appreciation of sycosis, an adapted character profile could be developed based on the combined personalities of the two. Two remedies were chosen for the syco-psoric comparison — Nat Mur and Nux Vomica.

With a foundation laid, the same steps for development conducted for syco-syphilis were applied to syco-psora. The selection of Nat Mur was a major leap, as many books refer to it as belonging to the sycotic miasm, but as will be seen the theme of syco-psora has quite a distinct and separate character which Nat Mur comfortably fits into.

It is by no means certain that our individual personality is the single inhabitant of these our corporeal frames ... We all do things both awake and asleep which surprise us. Perhaps we have co-tenants in this house we live in.

- Oliver Wendell Holmes

CHAPTER 9

Further Development of the Existing Miasms

We can see that by the time he came to Paris Hahnemann had considerably simplified his method of remedy selection. This was mainly because his ideas about the similimum had changed since the days when he intended it to cover the totality of the visible symptoms of the patient. Now, with a whole new theory of chronic disease behind him, he was determined to deal with the invisible symptoms too.

It is in the method of choosing the remedy for the patient that these casebooks manifest some of the most important discrepancies between the received information about Hahnemann's prescribing and the actual facts. Whatever Hahnemann might have thought and written in his early life, it is clear that in his later days he became a miasmatic prescriber ...

- Rima Handley

Further development into what already exists should have been a relatively straight-forward affair, but this was not the case. Because of the two new miasms, a reclassification of the main polychrests had to be done. Statistically, two-sevenths of our medicines had to be in an incorrect miasmatic group so an overhaul of all the major remedies was conducted.

In light of these new developments, remedies had to be reallocated from one miasmatic group to another deemed more appropriate. To allocate a remedy into a miasm based on pathology alone is incorrect, so also is to allocate on large and broad generals like < cold or > after sleep. To use < after sleep is more appropriate as it is less common but < cold is too general. Pathology never takes precedence over the mentals or generals in standard case-taking – why should it here?

Consider this quote in regards to reliance on pathology in order to understand disease given by Kent:

At the present day diseases are named in the books from their appearance and not from any idea as to what the nature or essence of sickness is, hence the disease names in our books are misleading, as they do not have reference to the sick man but to ultimates.

Practitioners understand that a single pathology does not make a case, this does not mean pathology should be ignored, but rather we should focus on the overall trend of the case, the repeated direction that these "ultimates" take. If someone gets a mouth ulcer, it does not mean they are entering into a syphilitic phase and to believe so is a mockery.

An overall essence and character has been developed for each miasm which was achieved for the existing miasms by comparing the traits of the major remedies from within each group. Sometimes this would be a general sensation like itching or dryness in the case of psora, but more often than not, these broader large rubrics would yield almost nothing of a discriminative nature. Smaller more unique rubrics such as "fear of poverty" were far more profitable for gathering more potentially psoric remedies. These smaller rubrics were selected from nosodes like Psorinum and Medorrhinum and were chosen as they help individualise and as such aid in a deeper understanding of the miasm. These nosodes were then compared with their major classical analogues such as Sulphur or Thuja, crossover symptoms were then repertorised to reveal any other remedies that may have this symptom. These new remedies were then measured against the other general and mental features. They must also be consistent with the essence of the miasm.

Even a sheet of paper has two sides.

- Japanese proverb

CHAPTER 10

Colour Coding the Miasms

Judging by everything that can be discovered about Hahnemann's miasmatic doctrine, all that was lacking to perfect it or, better still, to complement it – was some way to facilitate recognition of the characteristics of each miasm and, at the same time, to group the symptoms in a clinically useful way; so that this remarkable doctrine should not remain a mere subject of speculation, devoid of the formidable practical utility which it has to offer.

- Dr P S Ortega

As can be seen in *Chapter 7, The Number of Miasms*, the newly recognised miasms are named in accordance to their parental miasmatic origin. Hence the miasm which lies between sycosis and psora becomes the syco-psoric miasm. I understand that there are miasms being named in accordance with disease, the malarial miasm and the ringworm miasm being two examples of this. But I have decided against using a pathology as a descriptor for two primary reasons: firstly, as a student and now even more so as a teacher, I believe taking pathological names such as syphilis or cancer and using them as benchmarks no matter how accurate, is confusing as it is almost impossible for students and patients not to think of the actual diseases of syphilis or cancer. In homoeopathic terms it is not true to say that because someone may belong to the cancer miasm that there is cancer in the family. Nor can it be predicted that a person will get cancer, and lastly it most certainly does not mean that cancer is the only disease that belongs to that miasm. Cancer and syphilis are diseases that epitomise the character and potential that a particular miasm has, but it does not imply the actual disease.

The miasms were originally described by disease names because Hahnemann believed they were the result of actual infection. But the miasm theory has evolved immensely, and now a more complex and richer understanding of them exists. As many authors quite rightly point out, predisposition always precedes illness. If the predisposition were non-existent then the disease could not be acquired in the first place. In other words, how could one contract syphilis or tuberculosis without a preceding predisposition? Something had to create this physical susceptibility and this is why Kent stated that everybody must be psoric, yet not everyone displayed over-productive or destructive pathology, therefore if everyone was miasmatic that miasm had to be psora. To be accurate, the original miasm, psora, had to have more arcane origins otherwise the theory hit a dead end and could not explain itself.

Hence Kent regards psora as a spiritual sickness and writes, in relation to psora:

It goes to the very primitive wrong of the human race, the very first sickness of the human race, that is the spiritual sickness, from which first state the race progressed into what may be called the true susceptibility to psora, which in turn laid the foundation for other diseases ... Psora being the first and the other two coming later, it is proper for us to inquire into that state of the human race that would be suitable for the development of psora. There must have been a state of the human race suitable to the development of psora; it could not have come upon a perfectly healthy race, and it would not exist in a perfectly healthy race. There must have been some sickness prior to this state, which we recognise as the chronic miasm psora ...

The miasms are far more than a state of "never been well since". Therefore any disease allocated to them does it a disservice and hampers a true understanding of their nature. Parkinson's disease is a degenerative illness and syphilis is a degenerative miasm, but it is incorrect to make the claim that Parkinson's disease is syphilitic. It would be fair to say that the dominant miasm must have syphilis in it, but that means that this Parkinson's sufferer could belong to the syco-syphilitic, tubercular or cancer miasms. Miasmatic prescribing does not rest or fall on the proposal to eradicate the disease names, in truth it changes nothing at all in regards to its application, but I still think it avoids confusion and helps to clarify matters by not using pathological terms. It would also make life easier for our patients. Parents do not want to hear that their gorgeous little daughter is syphilitic or that their little prince is obviously cancer! It is far too difficult to divorce the miasm from the disease itself; this is the first and primary reason further disease names were decided against.

Secondly, for this model, colour coding rather than names was decided as more appropriate as it helps show miasmatic parentage and affiliation as well as its own unique miasmatic individuality in an easily understandable and recognisable way.

There are three primary miasms; there are also three primary colours. Therefore each one of these miasms could be assigned one of the primary colours that best suited that particular miasm's temperament. At this point I would like to acknowledge the work done by Dr Ortega in this respect and concede that while we have both decided to use colours as a way of describing miasmatic personality, and probably this is where the idea came from in the first place, I have used different colours for each miasm, so obviously our personal summaries of each primary miasm will be different.

For psora the colour yellow has been chosen. Yellow is warm and friendly, the colour of the sun, it is light, bright and welcoming. Yellow stimulates hunger and yellow is the colour of the liver.

Red has been given to sycosis. Red is hot and inflamed. Red is the colour of love, seduction and passion. Red is conspicuous and ostentatious. Red is jealous and revengeful; it is fiery and confrontational.

Blue was given to syphilis. Blue is cooling and deep. Blue is used to describe melancholy. Blues music howls with desperation and struggle, it sings of injustice and lost love. To quote: "The blues is about making a lot of other people feel bad, and making money while you're at it". Blue is soothing and tranquil while at the same time quiet and stationary.

Using these primary colours the coding for the mixed or complex miasms became a straight-forward affair. The beauty of colour coding a miasm is:

1. Miasms can be learned and remembered easily.
2. Colour coding highlights the unique character and feel of each miasmatic group.

3. Colour coding is a reminder that a number of miasmatic possibilities exist within in each case. For example if a patient is purple (syco-syphilitic) then they may display traits characteristic of this purple miasm, or they may display qualities of both blue (syphilis) and red (sycosis). Memorising the miasms by colour highlights the distinctness of each group while at the same time serving as a memory aid for the two groups it originates from.

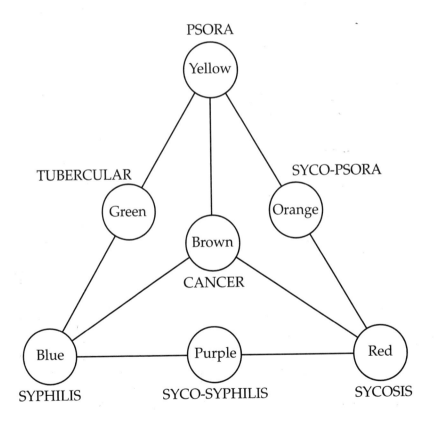

The colour allocation for each complex miasm includes:

1. Psora. Primary miasm. Primary colour – yellow.

2. Sycosis. Primary miasm. Primary colour – red.

3. Syphilis. Primary miasm. Primary colour – blue.

4. Syco-psora, mixed miasm. Complex of psora (yellow) and sycosis (red). Secondary colour – orange

5. Syco-syphilis, mixed miasm. Complex of sycosis (red) and syphilis (blue). Secondary colour – purple.

6. Tubercular, mixed miasm. Complex of syphilis (blue) and psora (yellow). Secondary colour – green

7. Cancer, mixed miasm. Complex of all the primary miasms, yellow, red and blue. Tertiary colour – brown.

In summary, the miasms have been colour coded for easy identification and to emphasise each miasm's unique individual character combined with a straightforward approach for recalling miasmatic origin. As an example, green (tubercular miasm) has a completely separate and unique character from either blue (syphilis) or yellow (psora). However remembering this miasm as green also makes it easier to remember that both yellow or blue facial features and symptoms can present themselves equally in any green case. From this point onwards the miasms will be referred to by their relevant colours.

The ultimate measure of a man is not where he stands in moments of comfort, but where he stands at times of challenge and controversy.

- Martin Luther King Jr

CHAPTER 11

Facial Features as Indicators to a Miasm

...the treatment of many chronic cases, the anamnesis of which had before been erroneously attributed to psora, has received another form and far more certainty. Nevertheless it is on the other hand not to be denied that this circumstance has given an additional difficulty to our practice, as we have not so far any certain signs by which we can distinguish certainly the domain of one miasma from that of the other.

- C M F von Boenninghausen

So far the book has centred on behavioural patterns, circumstances and energy cycles, but this is only half the story of miasmatic prescribing. Just as important is the ability to evaluate certain facial features and to understand that what is on the outside bears a direct relationship to what is on the inside. The old adage, "You cannot judge a book by its cover", is not entirely accurate. It is true that you cannot tell a person's story just by looking at their face, but facial structure can determine with reliability their dominant miasm.

Although I have quoted this passage from J H Allen earlier in the book, I think it is fitting to re-examine it paying close attention to the author's inference:

How generally we see the landmarks of one of these chronic miasms stamped upon the organism. We see it in every feature and every physiological process; in the shape and contour of the body; upon the visual expression, the face, nose, lips, ears, mouth, upon the hair, its growth, lustre and general beauty or lack of it. We see it upon the skin in its colour or shadings, its local temperature, yes, we can tell the miasm often by a touch, by that response in our very inner being, the mental, the moral, even the spiritual, give us responses of its presence and of its influence.

Each miasm influences psychological and structural development with its own unique stamp. It is impractical to suggest that a particular disease is psoric but the person that developed it is not. Psora can only flourish and develop under psoric conditions. A psoric person does not wake up one morning feeling strangely syphilitic. If one's body structure is determined by the dominant miasm as Allen and others suggest, and one dominant miasm can be replaced by another, then appearance should noticeably change in accordance with this miasmatic power struggle, and yet nowhere do we ever see this happen.

There is only one possible explanation for this, miasms do not rotate. Only the single dominant miasm theory can explain why. J H Allen has sufficient confidence to make statements like the one above. Whichever miasm is strong enough to mould structure and behaviour is strong enough to repel all other miasmatic challengers.

Analysing facial features has always been somewhat derided for two main reasons

1. Facial feature identification has, in previous systems, attempted to be definitive.

2. Facial feature identification has, in previous systems, attempted to be predictive.

Homoeopathic facial feature identification differs from many other practices of face reading in that it does not attempt to either predict the future, nor does it try to attribute any meaning or attitude to any single feature. Whilst miasms have a theme, facial features do not, they are signposts that guide us to the dominant miasm. Their sole and only purpose is to help identify which miasmatic family a person belongs to.

With the facial features, the problem faced by Boenninghausen in the opening quote is eradicated. The miasmatic facial feature identification process allows a practitioner to clearly and concisely identify which miasmatic group their patient belongs to. With practice, this can be done with such certainty that should the patient's story contradict the facial features of the case then the facial features are to be taken as the most accurate and resounding signpost to the miasm.

Syphilis as a disease left an indelible imprint by disfiguring generations to come. So too does the miasm to which this disease belongs. All the miasms have the ability to alter and reshape the body otherwise they would be unrecognisable and harmless. If they do reshape and alter, then their mark should be distinctive. Miasmatic prescribing based on facial feature identification is far more accurate than pathology or biographies in distinguishing one miasm from another.

In reference to pathology, we have to firmly establish the notion that miasms are merely ways of describing trends of illness. The syphilitic miasm means there is a destructive trend.

In sycosis there is a trend of overproduction and inflammation whilst psora produces a trend of "hypo" or absence conditions such as a generalised dryness. As a consequence, a psoric person suffers from all the dry diseases; eczema, pleurisy, and some forms of arthritis. Pathology can be misleading, which is why all the master homoeopaths were wary of it. They accept the importance of pathology but they never let it govern their ultimate decision. The person that has the pathology is far more relevant than the pathology they have. In reference to the miasms the same rules apply. Pathologies may be helpful indicators but they are not decision-makers.

Boenninghausen once asked, "Is it possible that there should also be condylomata which, like some cases of gonorrhoea, are not really of a sycotic nature and in their essentials have nothing in common with it?" Here Boenninghausen puts forward the question because he is aware that in clinical practice there are some things that simply do not add up. Pathological signs and symptoms are not precise indicators of the miasm. Warts may be a sycotic symptom but they can also be found in remedies outside of sycosis. Pathological signs and symptoms are good confirmatory symptoms but they are unreliable primary guides.

The mentals and miasmatic themes, although more solid, also have the same problem as pathology, it is true they are more distinct and therefore more "core" but they are open to misinterpretation. Many times I have interpreted a symptom to mean x, when after further consultations it becomes quite obvious that the patient meant y. Miasmatic themes are subjective forms of analysis and therefore create a potential minefield of problems.

Pathology is inaccurate as it deals only with disease outcomes, not what created them. Facial features are objective, distinguishable and stable. Some interpretation is still required but only in regards to discriminating between eyes that are wide set or close together, whether when someone smiles their teeth fill the whole of their smile or is there space on either side of the dental arch.

Not every Arsenicum patient is fastidious and not every patient needing Pulsatilla is weepy. In the same vein miasmatic themes are helpful guides to miasm selection, but they are hardly the be all and end all. Just as repertorisation is designed to direct a practitioner to the relevant remedies in the materia medica, the purpose of miasmatic grouping via facial feature recognition is to guide the practitioner to what remedies should be considered, and what remedies can be disregarded.

Reading facial features and using them as miasmatic indicators, in theory, is a relatively easy task, however like anything else it takes lots of practice to perfect it. Like taking a case, the facial feature identification process is about the subtlety only experience and constant comparative reading can provide. Using the chart provided, facial feature identification soon becomes an important part of clinical practice, but more than this, it becomes a way of life, a procedure you will find yourself doing with every person you meet and every movie you watch. Soon you will begin to see the different miasmatic dynamics that influence the relationships of those around you.

Practise. Practise. Practise. Don't become too downhearted too quickly if at first everything seems to blend. Faces, like rubrics, will, with experience, begin to make themselves known as distinct and unique characters rather than being an indistinguishable grey and, most important of all, always remember: **ethnicity is absolutely immaterial to this method**. The same facial feature indicators apply regardless of race, creed or colour.

Our deepest fear is not that we are inadequate. Our deepest fear is that we are powerful beyond measure. It is our light, not our darkness, that most frightens us. Now we ask ourselves, who am I to be brilliant, gorgeous, talented and fabulous? Actually, who are you not to be? You are a child of God. Your playing small does not serve the world. There is nothing enlightened about shrinking so that other people won't feel insecure about you. We were born to manifest the glory of God that is within us. It's not just in some of us; it's in everyone. And as we let our own light shine, we unconsciously give other people permission to do the same. As we are liberated from our own fear, our presence automatically liberates others.

- Marianne Williamson
(used by Nelson Mandela in his inaugural speech)

CHAPTER 12

How to Use the Miasms in Clinical Practice

If we are honest with ourselves we will discover that we have superstitions stemming back for perhaps hundreds of years represented in the belief systems of our unconscious mind. We have fear systems relevant to generations before us. We have prejudices that do not really apply to us ... Prejudices have stemmed from primitive and ignorant days throughout the course of man's evolution and have been programmed into our unconscious minds. They now belong to us and we automatically respond to them at the unconscious level.

- J Goulding

The modus operandi of miasmatic clinical prescribing is quite simple. Miasmatic prescribing aids remedy selection in two important ways. Firstly an understanding of miasmatic themes will assist in the selection of the most appropriate rubrics while the facial features help in actual remedy selection.

There have always been certain rules to repertorisation, and there is a definite hierarchy of symptoms if correct repertorisation is to take place. Using Kent's method of repertorisation, individualising mental symptoms hold the most prominence.

These include the fears and phobias, desires and aversions, temperament and character, in short all of those characteristics that help identify individuality. Hahnemann talks of the PQRS symptom as being the most important diagnostic, again because of its unique quality, it quickly separates one remedy from all others. Symptoms have appropriately been classified into individual and common symptoms – common symptoms being so classified because they are found in most cases of the disease in question. They describe the illness but not the person that has it; that task is performed by the individualising symptoms. The common symptoms rarely, if ever, form the basis of selection for a remedy. Kent for instance teaches that should we begin our repertorisation with a particular (common) symptom our repertorisation will almost certainly fail. To simply look up and give a remedy based on a presenting symptom only may very well be easy but it is also untrained and generally unsuccessful.

Many cases are presented with no general and no mental symptoms – only the symptoms common to sickness. When a successful prescription is made on such symptoms it is scarcely more than a "lucky hit." It cannot be classed as scientific prescribing.

The rules of symptom prescribing are just as relevant to miasmatic prescribing. There are certain miasmatic themes as well as general features that are so common to a particular miasmatic group that it should under the normal rules of prescribing scarcely be regarded as a symptom due to its commonality.

For example dissatisfaction is a well-known mental characteristic of the tubercular miasm, so also is a fear or draw towards ghosts and the supernatural. All these two symptoms tell you, is that your patient is most likely tubercular. It is the same as looking up chilly, runny nose, cough and tiredness while trying to prescribe for a cold. If you select these common miasmatic symptoms as primary rubrics, the repertorisation will only provide you with the most proven tubercular remedies, notably Phosphorus. But the selection of Phosphorus means a generalised prescription for the tubercular state and as such nothing more than a generalised improvement should be expected,

By understanding what is common to a miasm a more thorough appreciation as to which symptoms are important and which are not becomes easier. Dissatisfaction as a rubric in a person whose facial features are tubercular is nowhere near as rare and important as it is in a person whose facial features display psora or sycosis, whereas jealousy in sycosis is not as prominent a rubric as it is in a tubercular case. Withdrawal under stress in syphilis is not as important a rubric as it is in psora. This does not mean that a generalised repertorisation will provide a remedy that will fail – it simply means that often only eighty per cent of the case will be covered as the specific rubric that is a key to the case has been overlooked.

CHAPTER 13

FAQS

1. How does this method differ from other methods of prescribing?

It differs because the miasm is the central point of the prescription. This is done in accordance with Hahnemann's last works of recognising the miasm as the single most important factor in a case. In reference to actual prescribing and rubric selection it differs very little. Repertorisation is done according to the same rules as is remedy selection in accordance with keynotes of a case and essence. The major difference is that the remedy selected must come from the same miasmatic family as your patient.

2. Is a facial feature a look?

No, a facial feature is a specific characteristic that is measurable by position, size or angle such as a nose or a chin, a look is a quality.

3. How can miasms be applied practically?

Their application rests in limiting selection to a smaller number of remedies from your repertorisation rather than being left with an extensive group from which a selection must be made and provided that your facial features have been correctly labelled, miasmatic prescribing ensures that your prescription will cover the miasm dominating the case.

4. What are the different views on what miasms are?

There are a number of differing views as to what a miasm actually is.

First, there is the view that a miasm has a biological origin, that is, a miasm is a disease that engrafts itself onto our genetic material from which it is continually transferred, some say indefinitely, while others say until the appropriate homoeopathic remedy is given.

Second is the belief that a miasm is any disease that has been driven inward and has engrafted itself via suppression.

Third is the view that a miasm is an emotional reaction or state.

Finally, a miasm is an inherited predisposition that lays the foundation *for* protection against disease rather than being a consequence of it (defense mechanism). It is a continuous, ever present force that binds with our character. Homoeopathic Facial Analysis is based on this idea of miasms.

5. Can you be more than one miasm?

Any individual can have more that one miasm in them but the combination of the miasms will form a single entity in its own right. Therefore someone may have both psora and sycosis in equal proportions but they would now be regarded as syco-psoric. Even the facial features themselves often show the presence of less influencing, dormant miasms. Hence a person's facial features may still be yellow (psora) even though they may have some blue (syphilitic) features. This shows that even if other miasms can be noticed only one will be dominant.

6. Can a mental picture be one miasm and the physicals another?

Yes. I have seen many instances where a patient will display a mental image of orange for example, yet have the destructive pathology of blue. In cases such as this, as always, the facial features will guide you as to the *real* influence behind the symptoms. REMEMBER – IF THE FACIAL FEATURES DO NOT MATCH THE MIASMATIC THEME, THE FACIAL FEATURES ARE THE BEST GUIDES AS THERE IS NO INTERPRETATION. THEY ARE STRAIGHTFORWARD AND *ALWAYS* CORRECT.

7.   Can you predict what miasm you or your children will be?

Perhaps, but I have not looked into this area in any great depth. I fully appreciate that nothing is random, so there must be some pattern but I cannot see it yet.

8.   Will you always be the same miasm?

Yes. The miasms remain constant, they do not change. The conscious mind may come up with various ways of modifying or appeasing them but their influence and presence will always remain stable. As in astrology an Aquarian may come in a variety of forms and expressions, but an Aquarian they are and an Aquarian they will remain.

9.   Does your nature change after a miasmatic remedy is given?

Because a remedy will often alter the way you look at a problem, it would be fair to say that after a remedy a more constructive you may emerge to replace the more negative one, but you can never become a person that is incompatible to your genetic make-up, you will always be you, so it's important to be someone you like.

10. Why doesn't the right remedy take away the miasm?

The miasms are your genes. Nature through homoeopathy has provided an opportunity for genetic improvement that otherwise may take lifetimes. You are here for a specific purpose, your character, your form – everything is the way it is because it was necessary for it to be that way. Nature would never allow that to be taken away on a whim. The miasm you have inherited is needed by you as a defense mechanism; hence the health can be modified but the miasm never eradicated.

11. Are you attracted to the same miasmatic group in a partner?

Some people are, although most tend not to be. Whether for reasons of behavioural compensation or for genetic balance, most people will be attracted to a partner from outside of their own miasmatic group. However this also requires a great deal of maturity from both sides if this is to be compatible, as this person will have a completely different way of viewing things to you.

12. Do miasmatic themes imply that all happy people are psoric while all creative people are tubercular, etc.?

No, in fact one of the major points I have learned via miasmatic understanding is that many of the clichés regarding remedies and people are incorrect. A yellow person can be just as creative as a green and so on. A green or a yellow person may make a fine actor, but if we were to add up all of the famous actors we may find a disproportionate number of brown or green as they are able to adapt their personalities to nearly every part. Brown can understand all aspects of behaviour because they have all the miasms in them; green because they are able to imagine the exact happenings and events in their mind. But this is not the same as saying all actors are brown, or green or that all brown or green want to be actors. As with all things homoeopathic, miasmatic prescribing requires a degree of subtlety and refinement if it is to be properly applied.

13. Why are miasmatic themes different to remedy portraits?

A portrait is an attempt to render a description or resemblance to a remedy that is easily recognisable in the patient by the practitioner. A miasmatic theme is a topic that presents itself disproportionately when compared to the other miasmatic groups. However like rubrics of a remedy all of the points in a miasmatic theme should not be expected to be present in a case. Burning is a major theme in Arsenicum, so too is restlessness or fear or fastidiousness, but it is not expected that all these will be present in a single case and certainly not in every case. The same common sense needs to be applied to the miasmatic themes. For example, money is a theme for yellow, but they can be frivolous with it or they can be miserly, they may want to acquire a lot of it so they can retire early or they may moan about the lack of it throughout the consultation. What is important is that the energy of money surrounds the patient.

14. Does this method of facial feature identification need to be modified according to race?

No, facial feature recognition transcends all barriers of race. Remember this is not about a look or appearance; it is a review of individual features in relation to width, shape and texture. Unless there is a race without noses, ears, eyes, or mouths this method can be applied to everybody.

15. How good is pathology as a miasmatic indicator?

The influence or importance of pathology in miasmatic prescribing is no different to standard symptom-based prescribing. The severity of the pathology can tell you a great deal about the vital force of the patient. The type of pathology – destructive, overgrowth, absence, etc. – also imparts crucial information. But as always, it is the nature of the disease that is important, not the name. The most accurate indicator of the miasm is the facial features and their dominance.

16. Does pathology always fall within a certain miasmatic group? Is schizophrenia, for example, always syphilitic and warts always sycotic?

Warts are found in Aurum and Fluor Ac. They are also found in Hepar, Psorinum and Sulphur, indeed warts are found in a number of remedies from a number of miasms, so it cannot be stated that they indicate the presence of red as the *dominant* miasm. However it is true to say that the nature of overgrowth is displayed in warts and as such should be taken into consideration along with the other generals of the case. Likewise, pathologies such as Parkinson's disease or schizophrenia most likely have a blue influence. Therefore pathology in regards to understanding the disease process is an invaluable diagnostic tool as someone who has Parkinson's is not absolutely but certainly far less likely to be purely yellow or red. But this still means that a patient with a pathology such as this can be purple, brown or green, they don't have to be purely blue. Understanding this means that greater attention needs to be paid to all the remedies that contain blue*.

17. If someone in the family has had cancer does that mean everyone belongs to the cancer miasm?

No, in fact brown may not even be the dominant miasm in the person who has cancer. Case after case has shown that cancer in the family does not mean a dominant cancer miasm but it certainly draws attention that way if it is a continuously repeated trend. Cancer is found just as commonly in other groups as it is in brown. Parents, children and siblings often don't look alike or act alike or even have the same interests. I have seen families where nearly every member in it belonged to a different miasmatic group. On the other hand I have also seen families where only one parent may differ and the influence of one side totally outweighs any contribution from the other.

18. How do you know if there is a dominant miasm within a family? Does that mean your patient automatically belongs to that same group?

There is always a dominant miasm within every individual but the same cannot be said for entire families. Often people will take on the dominant miasm from a grandparent more than a parent. Why this is I cannot explain but it seems to be a relatively common phenomenon.

19. Will you always see the same facial features for each person within a miasmatic group?

Think of facial features like letters of the alphabet, even though there is a limited number, the variation of meanings, words and sentences made from them is endless. All the miasms have distinctive recognisable facial features, but their potential arrangement is infinite. There are millions of different looks, but if a person's yellow features outweigh all influences by other miasms, then that person is yellow.

*Footnote 2008 - This answer is based in the historically accepted concept that syphilis is the most destructive miasm. Clinical experience does not validate that syphilitically dominant people or people from miasms with a component of syphilis in them have a greater likelihood to suffer schizophrenia than people from other miasms.

20. How do you know which remedies fall into which miasmatic group and why?

All the miasms have some distinguishing qualities about them.

Blue, for example, has a tendency to withdraw. They can have high energy or they can have depression. Blue has themes of ulceration, degeneration, yellow/green discharges, they are aggravated at night and so on, and these symptoms build upon one another until an expression of the entire miasm begins to show itself. Once a miasmatic theme is established you have a 'genus epidemicus' around which remedies can be matched and grouped. Once a genus epidemicus has been arrived at for every miasmatic group, all remedies by virtue of their symptoms and essence can be categorised into their respective miasmatic family.

21. Why is the miasm the origin of all chronic disease?

Hahnemann believed that a miasm was behind all chronic illness. As such a miasm can be interpreted as a genetic blueprint determining strengths, weaknesses, mental outlook, inherent skills and disease propensity. To some degree chronic disease treatment or constitutional prescribing is like an extension of Schusslerism. This is the idea that if a cell is perfectly nourished, then there is no foothold for disease to enter. But these footholds do exist and what's more they repeat themselves. Observation also shows that these footholds run in families. A miasm is the conceptual name given to these footholds; if the miasms did not exist there would be no disease either in body, mind or character.

22. Why does this model say there are only seven real diseases?

Hahnemann stated that the miasms were the cause of all chronic suffering; all the different diseases that exist in the world are merely expressions of that miasm. In the end the three primary miasms of too little (yellow), too much (red) and perversion or destruction (blue) or the various combinations of each, are the only ways a disease can express itself. Every illness falls into one of these variant categories. Seven is the outcome of combining all three miasms in all their combinations. The miasm not only determines what type of pathology one is susceptible to but how far it is likely to progress. Take away if or how far a disease is allowed to develop and you take away the power of the illness. How circumstances are dealt with, the general environment determines what potentials will manifest, so free will plays an enormously important role.

23. Why will the miasm influence everything that happens in our lives?

A miasm is an energy and as such it will attract similar energies towards it. If it is a violent energy then it will cause violence in the person in whom it resides as well as attract and create the circumstances for violence to occur either to or around that person. Therefore we can say that a person who suffers violent and cruel things is just as influenced by a violent energy as those who inflicted the violence.

24. How do you know when a remedy has worked?

A remedy has worked when the patient feels better within themselves, they are sleeping soundly and waking refreshed, the ups and downs of daily life are being coped with and not exaggerated or denied, there is a balanced appetite for both food and physical output, defecation and urination are regular and the presenting physical symptoms that brought the patient to your clinic in the first place are going, gone or greatly reduced, relationships are cordial and emergencies and accidents are infrequent.

25. Can you transfer a miasm to another person?

This miasmatic model is based on genetic transference therefore each miasm is inherited. It is not a contagion that can be acquired from an outside source or person.

26. What happens if you give a well-indicated remedy but it's the wrong miasm?

This is most probably where the concept of "layers" came from. A remedy seemingly well indicated, fails to allow the patient to return to full health or still leaves them prone to accidents, trauma or chaos showing that the energy around the patient has not truly changed even though their symptoms may have been alleviated. If the true constitutional was found the patient would not be returning in a month's time with a new set of ailments. Many times a patient may return with their ailments diminished or gone, but their energy is no better, another sign of the right symptom similimum but the remedy does not fit the miasm. Sometimes a remedy can be given that perfectly fits the presenting symptoms but not the miasm and eighty per cent of the symptoms will diminish or go; this is fine if your patient is happy and it is still an extremely good prescription, but Hahnemann focused extensively on the miasms for a reason — he believed they were what kept the fire of disease burning. While a prescription made on symptom totality was good and valid, he believed that a prescription which included both symptoms and the underlying miasm was even better.

27. How do you know you have the miasm wrong?

The energy of the patient hasn't changed. As mentioned in Question 24, a remedy should change the symptoms and the energy and quality of the patient.

28. What happens if you give the wrong remedy but have chosen the right miasm?

Choosing the incorrect remedy whether based on symptom

prescribing only or symptoms and the miasm, is irrelevant, as the incorrect remedy is always the incorrect remedy regardless of its basis. As with any incorrect remedy, the two most likely outcomes are:

1. There may be an aggravation.

2. Nothing occurs at all.

29. Does miasmatic prescribing change the way I take a case?

No, the fundamental rules of case taking still apply. Miasmatic prescribing is an adjunct to conventional techniques not a replacement. In repertorising a case, however, there may be some minor changes, for example, often not as many mental symptoms need to be repertorised as many of them are just further examples of the miasm itself. It is not the genus epidemicus symptoms we are looking for but the individualising ones. In the same way many of the mental symptoms will be part of the genus epidemicus of the miasm and should be treated as such, this places greater emphasis on the importance of the generals. In a standard miasmatic-based repertorisation of six or seven rubrics, an average distribution of rubrics will include two to three mentals along with three to four generals.

30. What happens if I see more than one miasm in a patient's face?

Miasmatic facial feature identification is the same as taking rubrics for a case. In every case there will be symptoms that do not belong within the sphere of the remedies' action. However if the overall essence is Arsenicum then that remedy will clear all the symptoms regardless of whether they were found in the remedy or not. It is an overall dominance that we are looking for when selecting a remedy and it is a dominant miasm we are searching for in the facial features. There will be in most of your patients some red or blue, but if there is clearly more yellow, then psora is the dominant miasm and a yellow medicine must be selected. Like repertorisation itself, miasmatic prescribing is a numbers game with the art of essence and experience thrown in.

31. What happens if I can see half of one miasm in the face and half of another?

Then the patient in front of you most likely belongs to the complex miasm of the two presenting primary miasms. If you are seeing an equal distribution of blue and red then this patient is purple.

32. How long does it take to become good at this method?

It takes time to be good at anything worthwhile and miasmatic prescribing is no different. However its principles are simple and once some experience is gained it can be used with accuracy fairly quickly. However much of facial feature identification is a matter of degree and it is gaining this finesse that takes experience. Miasmatic prescribing will become second nature, but until it does, like all things it must be worked at.

33. Does miasmatic understanding have any bearing in a pathological prognosis?

If a patient presents with a diagnosis of cancer or any other progressive life threatening illness, there is no doubt that the less blue is in the picture the greater the chances of recovery. Yellow attempts to eradicate, red attempts to contain but blue is about concession. Blue is in damage control and attempts to minimise harm. Hence the more blue the harder and faster the remedy needs to work — the catch is the more blue there is, the less vital force we have to work with. This is the reason pathology was allowed to progress so far. Blue is destructive – that is its nature – the more blue, the worse the potential prognosis*.

*Footnote 2008 – The degree of pathology, the prognosis of the pathology and the strength of vital force within a patient DO NOT relate to any of the seven miasms. The syphilitic miasm (blue) suffers no more or less than any of the other miasms. 200 years of homœopthic literature indicate the above is true but as I analyse more patients via their facial structure alone I have not seen a relationship between any particular miasm and the degree of pathology. When I wrote this passage in 2002 I was still swayed by the relationship between the miasm and the type of disease suffered by the patient. The miasm is an indicator of how the body reacts and fights its own stress state once disease is established. Each miasm fights in its own specific way. Each of these seven responses to internal stress is enhanced by the introduction of the correct miasmatic remedy.

34. Do the miasms play a role in mental illness and prognosis?

There are certain areas of the body where each miasm seems to have a natural affinity, the GIT and the skin in yellow, muscles and female reproductive system in red and the bones and brain in blue. Therefore any deep mental illness has a likelihood of some blue involvement and again the more blue there is, the longer it takes for a remedy to have any influence. Understanding this helps qualify expectations. For example, treating someone with depression who is blue, may require more frequent administration* of a remedy than someone who is red. A yellow may with the aid of the right remedy or remedies emerge from their depression quickly, but to expect this with every case of depression or think you have chosen the wrong remedy when it does not happen, is to misunderstand the miasms. In depression blue may slowly revive and quickly slip back, whereas yellow may quickly revive and slowly slip back. Miasmatic understanding is a tool that helps a practitioner guide and manage a case.

35. Does a person resonate to a particular remedy with each group?

This is the age-old debate regarding constitutional remedies – do you stay the one constitutional remedy or do you change? My personal belief is that you change; otherwise the given remedy would not have done anything. However, in saying that, I have also seen many cases where a patient may continually need the same remedy over and over again, each dose working quickly and effectively. Because I don't have any firm beliefs as to which is right or wrong I have placed less pressure on myself. If I achieve what is expected with one remedy, then that is a good result. If I achieve what is expected through a series of remedies then that's a good result too. As long as both my patients and I are happy with the outcome, I give scant regard as to whether I got there by one remedy or ten – although one is always nicer.

36. Why are the miasms colour coded?

Colour coding breaks the concept of actual syphilis or cancer, etc. Once the concept of contagious disease is out of the practitioner's mind, they are free to understand the miasms for what they really are – an energy or force which ensnares people into believing erroneous ideas about themselves and others combined with a propensity towards the development and progression of a disease in accordance with this misbelief. Colour coding also assists in recognising each complex as containing elements of its parentage while at the same time accentuating its own individuality.

*Footnote 2008 – Further experimentation with posology has led me to favour a frequent daily dose (low potency – 6C or 30C) for all patients regardless of miasm or pathology. The more I understand homœopathy the more I realise it is an energy model and daily doses of the correct miasmatic totality remedy are beneficial to all patients suffering with stress and/or pathology.

37. Do any of the miasms resemble each other?

Yes, in fact often the opposite miasms will resemble each other. To explain, yellow can often resemble purple in many of its themes, however their drive will always be different. Like inimical remedies, miasmatic opposites often share the same outcomes or goals, but their generals and motivations remain distinct. Yellow and purple share common themes regarding immaturity, sex and money, however, what each is trying to achieve and why is distinct. Orange and blue share grief, trauma, violence and lost love. Red and green share excitement, purpose, passion and stimulation. Despite this similarity, each has a quality and flavour that distinguishes it. Sometimes, however, even this can be a mere shadow; this is why facial features are so important to master as they will always decide the case. Whether these opposites will attract each other I cannot say at this point, but it seems plausible.

Brown, in accordance with its nature because it contains all colours, can look like and get along with all groups.

PART TWO
MIASMATIC THEMES

Themes must be used with subtlety and wisdom. If misunderstood they will do more harm than good; if used appropriately they will provide assurance and confidence. FACIAL STRUCTURE WILL ALWAYS SUPERCEDE THE INTERPRETATION OF A THEME.

Emphasis is placed on the negative aspects of each colour because these are the conditions we are trying to treat. A more balanced perspective including the positive aspects of each colour group (miasm) can be found in **Soul & Survival** (2008)

Note: The people who make up the cases in this book are not represented in the photo section. To guarantee anonymity all photographs are of volunteers for the specific purpose of aiding in the production of this book.

CHAPTER 14

Miasmatic Themes - Psora (Yellow)

It required twelve years for Hahnemann to discover and gather together the evidence upon which he came to his conclusions. When a patient came to him who manifested chronic disease in any way he took pains to write down carefully in detail all the symptoms, from beginning to end, with the history of the father and mother, until he had collected a great number of appearances of diseases, not knowing yet what the outcome would be; but after this careful writing out of the symptoms of hundreds of patients, little and great, and comparing them and then gathering them together in one grand group, there appeared in the totality of this collection a picture of psora in all of its forms. Up to this time the world had been looking upon each one of these varying forms as distinct in itself ...

J.T. Kent

Miasmatic themes are wonderful adjuncts but, like the symptoms of a remedy, one should not expect to find all of them in each patient. There are thousands of separate symptoms for Sulphur, but very few of those symptoms have what is special enough to become a keynote symptom. A miasmatic theme is similar to keynote prescribing. Both are trying to define the most common life scenarios and patterns of behaviour any given miasm is likely to exhibit. They attempt to be guides not characterisations; therefore I am not saying this is what you will see, just to be alerted to this particular miasm if you do. As with remedies no single symptom or theme is strong enough to stand on its own, burning does not make you think of Sulphur alone. But with burning now add itching with a voracious appetite and quick explosive temper and now Sulphur becomes more obvious. Themes are no different to single symptoms, in order to be used effectively they must be in combination with other themes, facial structures and generalities, then and only then can a decision be made. Any decision made without all of these factors is little more than a guess. It is not expected that a patient will walk into your clinic displaying dozens of Sulphur symptoms and the same should be applied to themes and facial features. Very few patients are going to have all psoric or all sycotic facial features. Just as Sulphur has ulcers or warts but it is still psoric so each patient will display facial features that will show the presence of another miasm. Make a note of each *prominent* feature and place it in its appropriate miasmatic group; at the end tally them up and you should have your answer as to what miasmatic group your patient belongs. If the theme matches you can now understand your patient's drives and motivations more clearly. If the themes differ from the facial structure then the facial structure *always decides the miasmatic group*

WORK AND BUSINESS

Yellow often talk of work and business giving the impression that outside their immediate family, business is the most important thing in their lives. In this respect it can resemble both green and orange, yellow of course being the common denominator of the two. Work is important as it gives yellow a sense of self-esteem and provides a social meeting place, but most of all it is a way of making money. Yellow is wily and quick to assess the rules of the workplace. They sum up office politics and quickly understand who can be trusted and who cannot. Work also supplies social status, another important yellow requirement. Work gives position and wealth and yellow takes both of these very seriously. They can revel in their perceived power and at times exercise it indiscriminately.

While business is important, it does not automatically entail their undivided loyalty. Yellow will be as loyal to the company as the company is in rewarding them. Yellow is a survivor, they are the longest living of all the miasms and what is true of the physical always has its counterpart in the mind. Yellow not only survives, they soon flourish and profit. They love a happy workplace and enjoy the friendships they make, but at the slightest hint of exploitation or lack of respect they can easily leave for greener pastures. Yellow does not work for the fun of it, regardless of how pleasant the work place, there are better things they can be doing with their time, so if they have to drag themselves into the office they expect to be fully compensated for it.

Work for many is a way of achieving and maintaining a lifestyle rather than a desire to contribute to an art or science. They may make good hobbies but business is about money making. It would be even better should this occupation be of service to the community, but the "something that helps people" is less evident amongst yellow than it is with some of the other miasms. They can be strongly career-minded and ambitious, driven toward their goal.

Anxiety and pessimism regarding the future are deeply ingrained traits whether consciously acknowledged or not. The future does not take care of itself, it is something that must be prepared for in the present, if not, it may be bleak. It is a cold hard world and one must be able to look after oneself. The 'saving for a rainy day' or the 'being prepared' philosophies are good examples of yellow.

A fear of poverty or a desire to make a lot of money is a common driving force of yellow. They take their jobs or professions very seriously and they may be ruthless in order to get ahead. Another strong yellow theme, "a fear of social or business failure", also plays its part in the yellow desire to achieve. They can be irritable and quick tempered wishing to get the job done, but they bear little if any grudge and once the explosion is over they expect everyone and everything to return to normal.

Rather than risking everything in some profit or loss venture, yellow are more likely to play it safe, especially when it comes to money. A common yellow tale is of stable employment combined with some property interests and perhaps a business or two. Now the risk is evenly spread, that way if one venture should fail then all is not lost.

Yellow is constantly thinking, coming up with a variety of plans and ways to secure their future and make them 'a few bucks'. This is the constant theorising and making of many plans epitomised in Sulphur. Yellow is an entrepreneur whose fingers can be in a hundred different pies, a person who can make a go of anything, not always confident but always competent, yellow is pioneering stock, a salt of the earth pragmatist that is community minded, fair in their dealings and a hard worker.

Practicality being this type of yellow's strong point makes them perfect for the solutions based world of business but like a fish out of water when it comes to romance and relationships.

The nature of their job or the type of businesses they run, is immaterial, as many are not looking for a vocation. This bears a similarity to purple, but differs in that yellow want to become wealthy so they can retire early and be free to do the things they want to do. Purple may go on amassing wealth and power. Yellow are lifestyle motivated not power based.

MIND; IDEAS; abundant, clearness of mind; evening.

MIND; THOUGHTS; rush, flow of; evening.

MIND; FEAR; poverty. MIND; AVARICE.

MIND; BUSINESS; aptitude for.

LAZINESS

In direct contrast to the industrious yellow is the more indolent type. In many ways completely the opposite of their busy sibling but still assuredly yellow. This yellow propensity for laziness or indolence is most noticeable in any task or chore that is burdensome or unprofitable There is no doubt that everybody works better in a situation where the job at hand also happens to be enjoyable or profitable, but for yellow there is no other point, anything that does not have at least one of these two elements is a waste of time.

Psora is yellow like the sun, and, just like a beautiful sunny day they wish to enjoy and make the most of it, to socialise and revel in the things that make life worth living. Their plan is to get on and enjoy life as much as they possibly can in a warm, safe and friendly environment. To yellow the happiness and social contact provided by the workplace is more important than the job itself. Simply wanting to be social, work can be viewed as something that gets in the way of a nice lunch break with friends. Yellow wants the pay cheque, it's the work they have to do for it that's a problem. Of the two evils, avarice and laziness, avarice will always win out, so yellow will reluctantly comply with the rules of society and work, besides many yellows, no matter how unmotivated, could not bear the social stigma of long term unemployment, This type of yellow works because they have to.

Some, as earlier mentioned, have ambitions to retire early so they can fish, be more social and play tennis. None of this "slaving your guts out rubbish". Life is too short to be spent in an office or looking down a microscope. Playing golf, a few drinks, coffee and cake with friends, this is the meaning of life for yellow. Lacking the direction provided by motivation some yellows can drift their whole lives uncertain of what they would like to do. A capricious and changeable mind is a strong yellow signpost.

MIND; INDOLENCE; aversion to work.

MIND; BUSINESS; averse to.

INTIMACY AND EMBARRASSMENT

Relationships are where yellow feel the least comfortable. Yellow crave company but not necessarily a relationship. A relationship and a desire for company can become interchangeable terms, not wanting to be left alone but not particularly wishing to commit to deep intimacy either. To yellow a partner is someone you can rely on, they pitch in and help, they give comfort when the going gets tough and they offer protection and support personally and financially, there may or may not be any mention of love. Everything about yellow is practical and pragmatic. Neither highly intellectual nor highly emotional yellow have a down to earth common sense that enables them to deal capably with anything that comes their way.

Rarely is yellow the initiator behind a marital breakup. Intimacy is not one of yellow's strong points and as a consequence they can survive well in a relationship that others might consider functional, indeed yellow may even promote this functionality as it is more convenient to them, hence if the passion fades in a marriage often the last one to realise it will be yellow as they never regarded it highly or promoted it in the first place.

There can be a self-centredness, they do not want to be inhibited or restricted in any way, they can be loyal, even supportive to an extent, they can love you even though they are not demonstrably loving, a competent partner but an embarrassed lover. This is part of the selfishness of yellow, giving to others only in a fashion or to an extent that they feel comfortable with regardless of the needs of their partner. Consumed with their own day, they can sometimes forget about those around them.

Yellow can have a naivety and immaturity about sex. They will try and be mature about the subject but their eyes will be darting everywhere as they shift and shuffle in their seat, their discomfort obvious. They may mention the word sex, in lowered or hushed tones. Many times I have heard it referred to it as 'that area'. They may enjoy sex, but it is not a major priority and certainly not a drive. Their libido can be low, many will say 'I am just not that interested'. Yellow can also be very prim and proper and as such sex may be viewed as something vile, an embarrassing part of life used for procreation only. Consider the following rubric: MIND; AVERSION; sex; opposite, to; religious aversion to: puls., lyc., sulph. Only three remedies in total and all of them yellow. This can be seen in males as a mental aversion or as actual physical impotence, and in females as a mental aversion, vaginismus or strong thrush symptoms that either prevent or make intercourse uncomfortable.

MIND; AVERSION; sex; opposite, to; religious aversion to.

MIND; AVERSION; sex.

THE SURVIVOR

Yellow has great survival skills. They can seemingly get along with most people; they socialise well and have lots of friends. Yellow is a person whom "the system" benefits. Modern life can offer great rewards to those prepared to play by the rules, and yellow is ready and willing to comply. They are the fox of the human world adapting themselves to the demands of their environment and doing what is necessary to profit and flourish. Business and congeniality are amongst yellow's strongest attributes making them the ultimate networker.

One of their major character flaws is irritability. It may be a storm in a tea cup, or forgotten as soon as it is over but to others they can be perceived as grumpy or pushy. Always trying to get along with others many have learned to curb their irritability by counting to ten, others do it by counting to one thousand. Intolerant of mistakes, some can seem almost impossible to please. Yellow can be home bodies not needing to travel too far from home as they can find their enjoyment under their own roof. As a consequence yellow can be very house proud.

MIND; UNGRATEFUL.

MIND; IRRITABILITY.

BRAGGING AND EGOTISM

Placing emphasis on social standing and financial achievement, some will want to make sure as many people as possible are aware of their accomplishments. Finding themselves in a position of responsibility they may be carried away by their success. Yellow loves flattery. They have worked hard for the rewards of security and financial stability and now, self satisfied, some are happy to gloat.

> *MIND; BOASTER, braggart.*

> *MIND; FLATTERY; gives everything, when flattered.*

FAMILY AND FRIENDS

Along with business and finance, family and friends rank highest in yellow importance. Most can find just as much satisfaction inside the home as they can outside it. People can be an endless source of enjoyment for them. They enjoy their toys, boats, cars, stereos, but without friends to share them, they serve no purpose. They are comfortable with both small groups and large, yellow revel in the company and interaction of others. Some may place great emphasis on sport, they can have a competitive nature and they like to win, however they are rarely the "racket throwing" type. Sport serves as an outlet for the competitive side of their natures, but it is the social network a team sport provides that many like the most. Sport is a chance to get with your friends and have a common interest and some fun.

Some yellows, particularly the more material and security-minded, can be hard and demanding of their children. Their children may be at private school, regardless of whether the parents can afford it or not. Their children receive extra coaching and all of the trimmings yellow believe help guarantee their future prosperity and happiness.

The childhood family for yellow will remain one of the most influential forces in their lives. Often they are most alive and boisterous when in the company of their parents or siblings, only their children may ever hold as important a role. After marriage, particularly a yellow female – the males are often more interested in their careers or businesses – may have a problem cutting the umbilical cord when moving from the family home into the marital one. In contrast, for the more independent make a million by the time your forty type of yellow, home may be a restriction that they can't wait to escape.

Some may have problems relating to partners, but rarely will yellow have problems relating to friends. With coffee and small talk, yellow are in their element.

MIND; COMPANY; desire for.

GETTING ON WITH IT

Yellow has a strong ability to rebound and regroup quickly through ignoring or moving away from a problem. Yellow can dump what is worrying them and move on to happier things. Their tendency not to dwell or worry too much protects them from the emotional ravages and consequent pathologies other miasms have to bear. As one yellow patient in my clinic stated, "If it causes me too much worry then it's just not worth it so I drop it and don't think about it". "Ignorance is bliss"– whoever said these words was most likely yellow.

IGNORANCE

In the Buddhist tradition, regarding the negative emotions that keep people caught in the endless cycle of reincarnation, yellow would be ignorance. Yellow can fight to keep things the same, the responsibility that comes with knowledge can make life too complicated for this type of yellow.

Being happy where they are, "new" can disturb the equilibrium. Some yellows are unconcerned with responsibility, preferring to keep things light and fun. Knowledge can be seen as boring, something you have to acquire. Rather than valuable, it can be viewed as something that impinges and stops them from socialising. Yellow can lack emotional depth, rarely thinking outside of fun and immediate needs, some have never given themselves the opportunity to grow, and as a consequence find themselves ill equipped to relate to anyone except in a superficial way. Not surprisingly, they can be viewed as lightweight and naïve, a good time person who disappears when the going gets tough.

HELP AND GUIDANCE

When in trouble, the yellow instinct is to reach out for the help and guidance of others. Yellow rely on those around them to help them through situations they find too demanding. Yellow craves sympathy as can be seen with remedies like Pulsatilla, and rely on others to help them out, and in extreme cases are not averse to manipulating others to do things for them. Yellow need other people, as they give comfort, company and security. When in trouble they will contact people and seek reassurance, some may rely on others to make decisions for them.

Physically and psychologically the immediate reaction of yellow is to go outward. Remedies like Sulphur have a centrifugal action; every ailment that affects them will be thrown to the circumference, including mental and emotional problems. They must, by natural design, release themselves from a problem. The nature of yellow is to push out and overcome, physiologically yellow's vital force is driven to free itself. Perhaps this is why they have a problem with intimacy as it limits freedom? Yellow need an outlet; like their physical symptoms, their emotions and fears will be pushed outwards by the vital force so they can find vent, yellow cannot suppress, it goes against their nature.

Yellow need to talk, to express themselves and relieve the burden. This makes yellow perfect for self-help therapies. Addicted to discussing their emotional problems, as it is great social conversation, yellow can make themselves the perfect caricature of "all talk but no action". The quick and easy solutions offered by many new-age self-help theories only serve to pander to their "yellowness", and they can become so preoccupied in discussing their "issues" that the problem becomes lost. They may for a while seek counselling or become involved in a support group, but inevitably yellow will begin to feel trapped and bored and will wish to move on.

PESSIMISM AND HYPOCHONDRIA

Above all things, yellow has one major fear – the fear of being alone. Like all thoughts, the energy of it can be either positive or negative. In its positive form, the yellow fear of isolation can lead them to appreciate who they have around them. On the negative side, there are two major yellow conditions that will bring this fear to life, one is hypochondria, a condition that yellow is prone to, and the other is pessimism. Yellow can be terrible pessimists, never trusting life, they can become anti-change, stifling those around them until others, unable to bear their negative domination any longer, move away. For yellow their worst fear has now come to pass.

MIND; PESSIMIST.

MIND; DOUBTFUL; recovery, of.

RECOGNITION

An extension of this tendency to brag, yellow will often overestimate the efforts they have put in to accomplishing a task. Their streak of laziness combined with their desire for profit, means that some will go to extraordinary lengths to guarantee others recognise their contribution. Sometimes living off the past, it is nothing for a yellow to continually recount a time of hardship and effort in an attempt to show how 'shoulder to the grindstone' they can be. Making sure that they always get back the equivalent of what they give out, yellow will often 'just happen' to mention any good deed or extra effort.

YELLOW CASES

CASE-1 Mrs C L aged thirty three

Presented with postnatal depression, Mrs C L "cries a lot for no reason" and 'has a fear of coping'. Her depression comes on her like a cloud. She has anxiety attacks over her responsibilities. She just had her first child and began feeling depressed after her mother, who was staying with her to help out, left three months ago. Now she feels anxious, she panics, starts to cry, and becomes depressed. Her emotions are worse at night and her crying prevents her from sleeping. Her father died a year ago and she is still grieving his loss. She has rationalised his death but feels her grieving isn't complete. Her sister has been coming to help her as her husband works long hours, she hates being alone and needs constant company. Her sister arrives and immediately takes over minding the baby. This gives Mrs L an opportunity

to pour her emotions out to her sister. She has a fear of failing .
as a mother and expects too much of herself. Everything has
to be done perfectly. She has a dull aching in her stomach and
legs and she describes this as a 'heavy' feeling. She has stopped
breast-feeding as it made her feel worse. Sometimes the crying
is so bad it is uncontrollable. After crying she feels better. She is
always better when she has someone to talk to.

The rubrics chosen for her case were

MIND; COMPANY; desire for.

MIND; WEEPING, tearful mood; tendency; night.

MIND; CONSOLATION; amel.

GENERALITIES; HEAVINESS; internally.

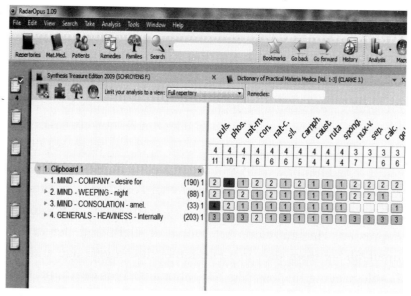

Facial features

Yellow

Bump on her nose

Ears slope backwards

Eyes down-turned

Strong lines under the eyes

Two front teeth are dominant

Red

Mouth is wide

Blue

Eyes are deep set

Mrs L has a dominance of yellow. The repertorisation shows that Phosphorus, Arsenicum, Camphor and Pulsatilla are high choices. Her need to have everything done perfectly may indicate Arsenicum but her face tells us Pulsatilla is a deeper miasmatic choice. I also wish to point out a number of yellow theme points. First she is better for company, and second her constant weeping makes her feel better. This shows the vital force continuously pushing outward. Any physical or emotional symptom will be pushed out in an attempt to try and heal itself. It is incorrect to suggest that all depression is based in blue. As this case shows, yellow can also suffer depression but rather than withdrawal and indifference the vital force of yellow still performs in an eradicating manner. Puls 10M single dose was given.

Two weeks later Mrs L reports that she has had no weeping at all. She feels much more positive and if occasionally anxious is able to get herself through without falling apart. Her sleep has improved and she hasn't felt depressed at all. She says she feels "100 per cent better". She enjoys the company of her sister but doesn't feel dependent on her.

Three months later she remains well and refers to this prescription as a "life-changing moment".

CASE 2 – Mr W B aged forty-three

Mr B presented with urinary problems and a white discharge from the penis. This has occurred for almost one year and he has had four courses of antibiotics that improved the condition momentarily but did not stop its continuous return. He experiences burning on urination and always feels a sense of fullness in the bladder. The urinary problem is much worse during the day but hardly bothers him in the evening or at night. The urine often looks dark but there is no odour. He is single and hasn't been in a relationship for a number of years. He says he has masturbated daily for most of his adult life. He works in a finance company and the hours are long and he is often tired at the end of the day. He has been diagnosed with candida by a naturopath on a number of occasions and his bowels are irregular. His favourite foods are starchy. When asked about being single he replies that he is unconcerned about relationships as they are too much work and prefers his life the way it is. There appear to be no emotional issues – Mr W B is a straightforward sort of person. When asked what he would like to see changed in his life he immediately answers "to get rid of this problem". In reference to the future his aims are "to get a pay rise and buy a bigger house".

The rubrics chosen for his case were

GENERALITIES; DAYTIME; agg.

BLADDER; FULLNESS, sensation of.

URETHRA; DISCHARGE; gleety.

URETHRA; PAIN; burning; urination; agg.; during.

URINE; COLOUR; dark.

MALE; MASTURBATION, disposition to.

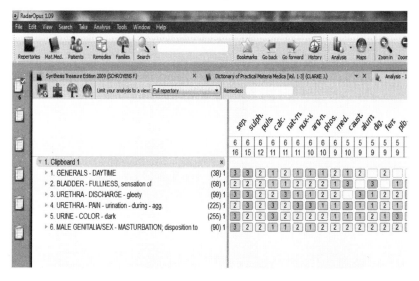

Facial features

Yellow

Bump on his nose

Ears slope backwards

Eyes down-turned

Eyes small

Forehead slopes back

Teeth don't fill mouth on smiling (compact smile)

Red

Lips full

Nose – ball shaped end

Blue

Eyes are deep set

Jutting chin (defined chin)

Mr W B has a dominance of yellow. The repertorisation shows Sepia most highly and also includes Medhorrinum. It is unusual for a nosode to come up so highly in a repertorisation and considering his problem Med. would have been my first choice prior to facial diagnosis. However as we are dealing with a yellow case it requires a yellow remedy. This leaves Sulphur and Pulsatilla as the only two remedies of choice. On questioning he mentions hot feet at night and being very overheated long after his shower. Sulphur 10M single dose was given.

Two weeks later he reports that his stools became normal within a few days. The discharge has reduced by 80 per cent and a urine test was normal. The bloating and burning have almost disappeared. Four weeks later his improvement has come to a standstill (20 per cent of symptoms remaining). Repeat Sulph 10M. One year later Mr W B returns again with the same symptoms. He states that he has been well since his last visit and all symptoms had completely disappeared. They have started to return in the last month. Sulph 10M is prescribed again and all symptoms improve within four days.

THE GENERALS OF YELLOW

SENSATIONS

Itchiness

Heat

Dryness

Roughness

Crawling

Burning

Bursting

One part hot while another part cold

Throbbing

Scalded

Drawing

Sensation as of a stone in the stomach

Easily gets lost

FOOD

Desires sweets

Thirstless

Worse for alcohol.

Worse for acids

Worse for coffee

Craves coffee

Worse for rich food

Worse milk and meat

Aversion to pork

Aversion to fatty food

Craves beer

Worse for onions

REPRODUCTIVE

Impotence

Breast lumps

Aversion to coition

Excess foetal movements

Amenorrhoea

Thrush

Erections with no feeling

Blood between periods

Easy conception

Male and female indifference to sex

Coldness of the genitals

Smallness of the genitals

Retracted testes

Delayed puberty in females

Feeble erections

Prostate problems

Weak erectile power

AMELIORATIONS

Summer

Open air

Warmth

Pressure

Eating

After sleep

Cold applications

Natural discharges

AGGRAVATIONS

Morning

Washing

Winter

Business failure

Coition

11.00 a.m./p.m.

Lifting

Uncovering

Fluid loss

Drafts

Lying on painful side

Overstrain

Riding

Driving

Periodically

Odours

Flowers

Standing

Stooping

PATHOLOGY

Varicose veins. Piles and **haemorrhoids. Heartburn** and reflux. Liver problems. Blood noses. **Thrush, eczema.** Cystitis. Low blood pressure and fainting. **Pleurisy, lumbago.** Rheumatism of the joints. Bed wetting. **Allergies, hay fever, cancer** and tumours. Obstructed nose. **Irritable bowel,** aches. Migraines. Sneezing. **Over reaction to allopathic medications** and over reaction and allergic disturbances generally. There can be rawness as a sensation. There can be heat, red streaks, poor reaction, easy sweating, and foul discharges. It affects the **palms and the soles**. Discharges acrid. Alternating complaints. **Alternating symptoms.** Flatulence well before the attack. **Liver and Gallbladder** symptoms. Headaches from concentration. Wrinkled and dry skin. 11.00 a.m. Worms. Localised oedema.

CHAPTER 15

Miasmatic Themes - Sycosis (Red)

POOR MEMORY

There are very few red people that do not have a problem with their ability to think. Whether in writing or talking, most have a problem communicating effectively. Unlike their green cousins who talk freely and easily, red can become tongue-tied, shy and defensive. Recall is limited when under pressure; they only realise what should have been said after the moment has passed, some because they have a thousand different thoughts all at the same time, whilst others can be totally blank, their mind in some far-off place. Red, guarded about their personality, or more precisely, their perceived lack of it, are busy trying to sum up what they think you want to hear, feeling this is the best method to make you like them. Many portray a character they believe others will accept more commonly than their own personalities until finally many feel trapped in an image they cannot move beyond.

With busy cluttered minds they often lose the thread of the conversation, their mouths talking about one topic whilst their minds are concentrating on another. This results in a confused mess of half-statements and sentences that trail off into nothing as their point gets totally lost. Information input is also scattered; not concentrating fully on the events around them, means only bits and pieces are being turned into memory rather than whole events, leaving many with just enough memory of an event to know that it occurred but not enough to make sense of it. Hence red often have an entirely different recall of events from others who were present.

MIND; MISTAKES, makes; talking; wrong; words, using.

MIND; MISTAKES, makes; talking; misplacing words.

MIND; ANSWER, answering, answers; slowly.

DAZED AND CONFUSED

To outsiders red may sometimes appear a little scattered, a person whose mind is jumping around restlessly. Some may come across as guarded and secretive, another defence to their instinctual belief that others disapprove of them, hence they keep their personalities secret and locked away. Lastly some come across as completely dazed. Someone who is not quite there, as if their body is here on earth while their mind is out exploring the universe. Staring blankly when questioned, their eyes can take on an almost 'out of focus' appearance.

Red has confusion about their identity, often borrowing a personality or manufacturing one they believe is more attractive or appealing. Only brown, due to the red component, is as big a personality mimic. Red may go through their whole lives with a manufactured personality. This serves the purpose of making them presentable as well as throwing others off the scent of their true personalities which they believe others would reject. The difference between red and brown in this respect, is that brown may lose themselves completely in the role, whereas while red will assume an image, there is always a part of them which recognises it for the act that it is. Brown may take on the role of the perfect mother, so also may red, but where brown will be successful, red may end up a portrait of Tyler's Sepia, ready to explode at the drop of a hat, sick of always having to do things they will get furious if taken for granted, their role or persona was designed to make them recognised and accepted not ignored, brown by contrast may be ignored but will still carry on regardless.

Red is torn in two, split down the middle by this charade. For many it has become a hindrance instead of a hiding place.

MIND; CONFUSION of mind; identity, as to his.

MIND; CONFUSION of mind; identity, as to his; duality, sensation of.

MIND; DELUSIONS, imaginations; separated; mind and body are

SEPARATE

Red believe they are different, a gulf exists that divides them from everyone else. They have a sense that if others really knew who they were, they would be repulsed by them. If they knew 'who I am' thinks red; 'what I really look like, what I really think and believe, what I like', no one would want me near them. Because of this, many put on an act, they are constantly on guard or just quiet and elusive. There are some that cannot keep this duality going; and as a result many choose to protect themselves by hiding their guilt or shame through introversion. To anyone outside of this miasm, the natural assumption is they must have something to hide, they have a secret, a reason for behaving this way, but this is the damage done by the miasm, it is an unjustified mode of thinking about yourself, that draws toward it the same energy it fears. Trying to hide themselves from others, those around them will either

a. feel less comfortable around them and so tend to socialise with other friends rather than red, isolating them even more and validating their notion that others don't like or accept them as much as they do others, or

b. because they are keeping a secret they may act secretively, which only serves as speculation that they have a secret.

Fearing judgment and embarrassment red can be shy and withdrawn, a far cry from the extroverted character some may expect to see as a display of sycosis. They can become uncommunicative, sullen and withdrawn. Red is about containment, containment of infection, containment of disease and containment of personality. Knowing that others think of them as strange or moody only serves to make them more so.

Separation is an example of detachment and this knowledge goes a long way to explaining the indifference so strongly present in remedies such as Sepia. Detached from others and detached from their environment, red is in a constant struggle trying to fit in and be accepted.

ALTERED STATES

Red can also be separated from others because of their lack of clarity and dreamy state of mind. As stated earlier many have a mind in which confusion reigns. Sometimes feeling as if they're not quite present in the moment, oftentimes described as an "odd disconnection" they can find themselves in a hazy, delirious type of state where everything can have a dreamlike quality. Some describe it as like being on drugs or having too much to drink or, as one patient stated, "It's as if there is a veil that lets me see everything that is going on but cuts off any real contact."

This dreamy, drug like state has, like all things, an energy of its own which entraps as well as attracts equivalent energies. For this reason red can be drawn towards drugs as a type of similimum, feeling at home and comfortable when either stoned or intoxicated; red can be drawn into a drug culture. This attraction is more likely to be towards drugs that give a calm 'spacey' effect rather than obliteration as this is closer to their similimum. There is a saying, that a person's true personality comes out after they have been drinking. This will be especially noticeable for red as they are, along with brown, the most compensated and suppressed of the miasms. After alcohol yellow may become social, green may become flirtatious, blue withdrawn, etc. But it is red and brown that can have a complete personality change.

Not all will turn to drugs or alcohol as their similimum to this strange disconnected feeling. Some will involve themselves in meditation, television or video games, anything that offers a virtual reality or altered state. Shamanic ceremonies, revivalist meetings, feel-good self-empowerment seminars, all are drugs in the context that they alter common daily consciousness and replace it with a state they would otherwise not feel of their own accord.

MIND; CONFUSION of mind; dream, as if in.

MIND; DAYDREAMING; tendency for.

MIND; CONFUSION of mind; intoxicated, as if.

STUPEFACTION, as if intoxicated; morning; rising, after. of.

MIND; MEDITATION.

WILD

Being confused or in a dazed condition, decision-making can be difficult. The tendency to make mistakes is high and the propensity to clutch on to anything as a quick means of stabilising oneself is common. This makes red impetuous and grasping, it also makes them clumsy. They can make clumsy mistakes and clumsy decisions. Often not thinking things through, their whole life can be a series of patch-up jobs, constantly trying to make up for the problems caused by haste when patience was required. This can make them seem irresponsible and now, it seems in the mind of red, as if everyone is pointing the finger of blame at them, accentuating the suspicious side of their natures.

Irresponsibility can be a miasmatic theme of red. They make hasty decisions that seem a good idea at the time. They have a habit of blaming others for not making their wishes clear enough, thereby *causing* red to do something wrong. Blame is a strong feature of this miasm as it takes the attention off them. Being jealous and secretive often they will look for an excuse or scapegoat as to why something went wrong. Red has no hesitation at pointing the finger at someone else. Everything may always be someone else's fault. They can become jealous and envious of the achievements of others; in their eyes other people seem to do things effortlessly, while they always have to struggle to achieve the same result.

Having a wild whirling mind can serve to draw them into whirlwind lifestyles. Like the child who never wants to get off the roller-coaster, they are always on the lookout for the next area of stimulation. In complete contrast, the exact opposite can also happen, many needing peace and quiet to offset the frenzy in their head.

RESPONSIBILITY; aversion to.

MIND; IMPETUOUS.

MIND; DELIRIUM; maniacal) (wild) (Mania).

MIND; WILD feeling in head.

INDIFFERENCE

Indifference in this miasm plays its major role with sex and the family. Best seen in Sepia but also in Thuja, red can be asexual by nature without any instinctive inclination or by lifestyle as they throw all their energy into a career. However it should be pointed out that this is less common, as their general theme is one of excess rather than of absence. Usually it is their overabundant sex drive that will be causing more problems than their unwillingness to participate, nonetheless there is a percentage that are so desperate to lock themselves away and go unnoticed that the last thing they want is to be on call for the needs of a partner or family.

MIND; INDIFFERENCE, apathy; opposite sex, to.

MIND; RESPONSIBILITY; aversion to.

MIND; INDIFFERENCE, apathy; duties, to; domestic.

MIND; AMOROUS; disposition.

MIND; LASCIVIOUSNESS, lustfulness.

LOVE, BODY IMAGE AND SEX APPEAL

As some want to hide and go unnoticed others will yearn to be seen. Beauty is a prime driving force, whether in fashion, body image or sex appeal. A beautiful body takes many forms and the perfect body for one may be an abomination to another. Body building is a good example of this. Perfectly sculpted bulging muscles to one may be a sickening sight to another, anorexia is another example of how one person can look in the mirror and say yes while another may view the same person and say no. Red have an ability to exercise their will and see things through, to focus on a particular objective and reach it. This is an expression of the rubric 'fixed ideas' found in many red remedies such as Cannabis and Thuja. "Fixed ideas" does not always mean obsessional thinking; it can also be used to describe stubborn determination.

Red can have the belief they are ugly, or at least not as attractive as they should be. Others seem prettier or more handsome making them feel left out. Red can feel they are the ones that only desperate people with no other options would choose. Fine delicate features are often revered as beautiful. Sometimes red features are broad and large. Acne, a common pathology of this miasm, can make teenagers feel ugly, spotty and undesirable. With such poor self-esteem, they will shrink into themselves and their body posture soon takes on the form of someone wanting to go unnoticed, making them less attractive and reinforcing their belief that no one is interested in them. Certain people are popular and have lots of admirers around them, some miasmatic groups will care little about this, but not red; jealousy is far too dominant and powerful an emotion for them to ignore. Some reds will try and buy love by giving their partners a slave, someone who will never upset them, do anything they want and wait on them hand and foot, only to be treated with disrespect and perhaps left for somebody else, confirming their "unlovable" view of themselves. Others may become promiscuous, buying love with sex or helping quell the notion they are undesirable by being desired by everyone. To be loved and desired is, for some, life's ultimate aim and they will do anything to guarantee they have it. Some may become sexually active early or marry at a young age. As they are both impulsive and in need of love, it is not uncommon for red to marry early, proving they are loved and desired, a decision many will regret later.

A few from this group will be forever bracing themselves for the day when their partner leaves them. Their partner may have no intention of this and may love them dearly, but that does not take away this feeling. An irrational miasmatic based fear cannot be rationalised away. Even years down the track red can wonder what their partner is *really* doing with them.

Others can deride the whole tradition of love. Marriage, the supposed ultimate symbol of love, can bear the greatest weight of this anti-love stance. Red may reject love and intimacy in all its forms, scoffing at people who adopt the "suburban ball and chain", prefer instead to stay career minded, focused and free. Angered at the shallowness of the world's inability to see beyond the makeup, they may decide to become a crusader against sexism, trying to eliminate gender and desire. Others can become asexual rather than antisexual. Deciding to live alone and have a simple and quiet life. Finding it grossly unfair, red may become infuriated when another is viewed as a sex object, or if people get promotions or gifts their talents or personalities don't deserve because of their looks, or when someone flaunts themselves and deliberately uses their wares to get what they want.

But to some from this miasm, beauty and sexuality are everything. Appearance is all that counts and everyone is judged and graded by it. Whilst our previous type was angry at anyone who was attractive, this red is ashamed of anyone who is not. It cannot be over emphasised how important it is for them to be found attractive, sexually desirable and loved.

Some in this miasm can have both sides of the miasm in them at the same time. They want to be loved and sexually desired, but at the same time become extremely embarrassed and want the ground to open and swallow them when they are.

Many are in love with love. Romance is the only thing that makes life worthwhile, they are real life Mills and Boon novels. Love is ecstasy, it takes them to another place and like the chapter on altered states, it is dreamy and exhilarating, as a consequence they crave to be "in love", another red similimum. No longer in the drug like ecstasy new love creates, they can sometimes feel let down, disappointed that this is all they are going to get. Again feeling left out, others find love and happiness, why can't I? It must be me.

MIND; INDIFFERENCE, apathy; opposite sex, to.

MIND; CHILDREN; aversion to.

MIND; SENTIMENTAL; moonlight, in, ecstatic love.

MIND; ECSTASY.

MOODY AND BROODING

Red are extremely emotional and as a consequence, weeping and emotional distress are common features. Hiding themselves, they may have a poker face that gives nothing away. Displaying few emotions their face is often smooth and wrinkle free as they age making them look much younger than their age or more attractive than many around them. Again we see the miasm at work, afraid of their sexuality and emotions red may display very little, choosing to remain cool and reserved. But to some this only serves to make them more mysterious and alluring. Suspicious of what others are thinking, they cannot be teased and often take things in bad part. They can feel sorry for themselves and have a feeling of being incomplete and sad until they find love.

SECRETIVE AND SUSPICIOUS

Because red is hiding themselves from others, their projection is that others have secrets also. Everyone keeps themselves hidden, no one can be trusted implicitly as you never really know what someone else is thinking. This is the cornerstone behind the suspicious nature of red.

Vermulen's synoptic repertory in reference to this suspicious nature states the following about Thuja:

They feel UNLOVABLE. They think that if someone knew who they really were they could not possibly love them. Because they feel they can never be loved they make an extra effort to be liked. They look around to see what is most popular, how they walk, dress, what they do, etc., to see what is successful. Then they go about IMITATING this systematically and scientifically, copying what they think works in the world and by adulthood they have the PERFECT IMAGE [Gray]. Feeling of UGLINESS inside. SELF CONTEMPT [perfectly hidden].

Outer appearance and self presentation become extremely important, leading to trickery, manipulation, deceit. "The great masquerader." Holds information back.

Being so guarded, red can become spiteful and vicious in their own protection, should anyone get too close to the mark regarding what is hidden inside. They will have no compunction in attacking to stop others in their tracks. Here red deserves its "mischievous" reputation relocating blame or perhaps getting in first by casting aspersions, Shakespeare in Hamlet once wrote: "The lady doth protest too much methinks". Subtlety sometimes not being one of red's strongest points, they may give themselves away by their vehement attacks. Becoming abusive and insulting, they can behave like the trapped animal they feel they are. Habits, desires and motives, all are hidden away in red.

MIND; ALCOHOLISM, dipsomania; drinking on the sly.

MIND; OBSTINATE, headstrong; declares there is nothing the matter with him; Well; says he is, when very sick.

SPACE, TIME AND OTHER DIMENSIONS

One of the last aspects I wish to cover is red's time and space sense. Red can be clairvoyant, being subject to many déjà vu experiences and with some, feeling or seeing spirits around them. Some speak of easy and frequent astral travel while others talk of prophetic dreams. Others talk of a "sense" they may frequently get, premonitions that life experience has frequently taught them to trust.

Red like purple can experience feelings of spiritual possession. However unlike purple, these feelings are usually transitory and cause only momentary discomfort; rarely have I witnessed someone from this miasmatic group believe themselves to be possessed. I have heard some talk of momentary loss as if another will was channelling through them, but never have I seen the type of long-term "possession" that resembles schizophrenia.

Time is another aspect that can be scattered and disorganised. Most characterised in remedies such as Cannabis Indica and Nux

Moschata. Red can feel outside of time and space, sometimes as if both were nonexistent, red can feel outside of them, unable to influence their will or even momentarily controlled by a stronger force than their own. Time often gets away from them and they have great trouble living with its restraints.

MIND; ANTICIPATION; matters, for, before they occur, and generally correctly.

MIND; DELUSIONS, imaginations; superhuman; control, is under.

MIND; DELUSIONS, imaginations; time; exaggeration of.
MIND; DELUSIONS, imaginations; footsteps, hears; behind him.

INTENSITY

Displayed in a variety of different ways, sport, business, sex, recreation, in their whole personality in general, red displays a force of will and intensity that spotlights a character that is extroverted and competitive, there is nothing red won't try and, when they do, they will do so with maximum effort and a minimum of inhibition.

They work hard and play hard as the saying goes, to some there are only two speeds in life; full on and full stop.

RED CASES

CASE 1 – Mrs R V aged twenty-six

Mrs R V presents with acne. She has had this problem since she was twenty-one and it is worse on her face, back and chest. Her acne improved slightly after the birth of her first child. Based on this her doctor prescribed hormonal medication but this made her skin worse. The skin on her face is oily but on the rest of her body it is dry. Her skin improves after sleep. She was under a lot of stress at the age of twenty one due to her forthcoming marriage. She has had sexual problems since the birth of her daughter, intercourse is painful and she has no interest in sex anymore. Mostly she tries to avoid her husband as she often feels angry when around him. She describes him as selfish and has problems with the way he puts his mother before her. She used to love going to parties but now doesn't enjoy it as much. She loves feeling attractive and enjoys dressing up and going dancing. She often does this with her friends, rarely her husband. Other men find her attractive and she enjoys their attention although her skin makes her feel less attractive. Recently she discovered that her husband has been unfaithful and she feels betrayed. Her description of herself is of a busy mother who is independent, determined and when pushed not averse to shouting. She works hard and does things quickly. There is a history of heart, kidney problems and arthritis in her family. Previously during winter she would have at least one bout of bronchitis. Her periods are painful and the flow is usually brown. With some cycles she feels nauseous and can sometimes vomit on the first day. Often her periods are irregular.

The rubrics chosen for her case were

MIND; BUSY.

FEMALE; COITION; aversion to.

FEMALE; COITION; painful.

FEMALE; MENSES; brown.

STOMACH; NAUSEA; menses; during.

GENERALITIES; SLEEP; amel.; after.

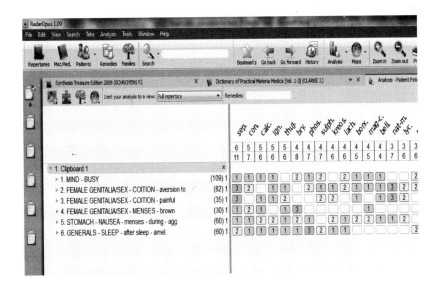

Facial features

Red

Straight hairline

Low hairline

Full bridge of nose on profile

Nose wide

Lips full

Single line between eyes

Teeth fill the mouth

Blue

Cheekbones

The theme in this case is all about attraction, appearance, dancing and jealousy. Her facial features had a dominance of red and a standard, orthodox repertorisation showed Sepia to be the major remedy. Sepia 200C was given. Two weeks later she reports feeling more happy and relaxed and definitely less angry.

She is not trying to do everything for everybody but allowing others to take over as required. Her face is less oily and starting to clear. Her pain during sex has diminished considerably. No further remedy is given at this point. Four weeks later Miss R V is beginning to slip back and is given Sepia 1M single dose. One month later she feels well and her skin has been clear for three weeks. Two months later Sepia 1M is repeated again as her symptoms have started to return – this prescription lasts for four months when Sepia 10M is given followed by a quick and positive result for another six months. She has no more period pain and the flow is red, there is no nausea or vomiting. Her skin is clear and there is no pain during sex. In general she is feeling happier.

CASE 2 – Mr P T aged forty-eight

His main problem is tachycardia, to the extent that every time he moves the problem commences and forces him to stop what he is doing. He has now become housebound and cannot work; he is a carpenter. He experienced chest pain and on three occasions was admitted to hospital. Tests revealed there was no organic cause for the palpitations or pain. His sleep is poor and he is constantly woken by heart palpitations, and suffers from terrible nightmares. He can't remember them in detail but feels restless most of the night. He has muscular soreness and has coldness in his left lower arm. Soccer is his love but he can no longer play the game. He has headaches every day and frequent migraines that begin with flashing lights in his vision. His wife died from cancer ten years ago and he still grieves for her. He often dreams of her at night. He has had this heart problem for the last eight months and is unaware of any extra stress that may have contributed to the problem. He has been given Nat Mur. by another homoeopath which had no effect.

The rubrics chosen for his case were

MIND; GRIEF.

MIND; DREAMS; nightmare.

CHEST; PALPITATION heart; motion; agg.

GENERALITIES; MOTION; agg. SLEEP; RESTLESS.

EXTREMITIES; COLDNESS; Forearm.

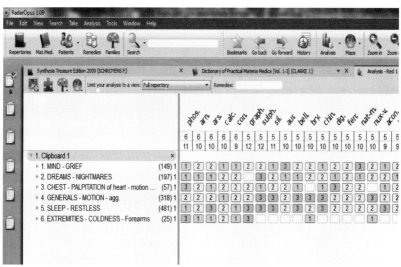

Facial features

Yellow

Forehead slopes back

Nose had a bump

Ears are sloping back

Eyes are close set

Red

Forehead – Full brow

Nose bridge is full

Nose is wide

Mouth is wide

Cleft in chin

Large gap between front teeth

Even teeth

Blue

Hair loss

Based on theme alone it is clear to see why Mr P T had been given Nat Mur. However his facial features indicate he is red not orange to which Nat Mur. belongs. Arnica was the only red remedy out of the first ten in his repertorisation. Arnica 1M was given single dose. Two weeks later he reported that his tachycardia had stopped within forty eight hours; his sleep had also improved. A very sore elbow that occurred alongside the tachycardia, not previously mentioned, also disappeared. His headaches diminished and he was able to get out and walk at a moderate pace without any problems. Four weeks later the headaches were beginning to worsen and he was starting to wake infrequently. Arnica 1M was repeated. One month later all symptoms including the headache are gone and three months later he remains well.

THE GENERALS OF RED

SENSATIONS

Ball

Numbness

Throbbing

Bruised

Constriction

Pulsation

Inflamed

Sticking

Stitching

Swollen

Crosswise direction

FOOD

Craves; acids, pickles, sour, vinegar, olives

Aversion; meat, potatoes, milk

REPRODUCTIVE

Fibroids

Retracted nipples

Abortion

Painful coition

Prolapse

Fish-brine odours

AGGRAVATIONS

Touch

Warmth/heat

Afternoon

Evening

Autumn

Jar

Suppression

Moonlight

AMELIORATIONS

Lying on abdomen

Motion

Cool air

Fanned/breeze

Stretching

Bending backwards

PATHOLOGY

Obesity. **Coccyx**. Spine. **Warts**. Inflammation. Meningitis. High blood pressure. Hips. Diarrhoea. Asthma. **Arthritis**. Oedema. Boils. Blisters. **Goitre** Abortion. **Infertility**. Prolapse. **Ovarian cysts**. **Fibroids**. Rheumatoid arthritis. Paralysis. **Injuries**. **Accidents**. Angina. Feet. Urticaria. **Acne**. Stroke. **Excessive hair**. Retracted nipples. Profuse discharges. Fainting. Gout.

CHAPTER 16

Miasmatic Themes - Syphilis (Blue)

DEPTH

Blue is deep. It is introspective and it is wise. They can have understanding and tolerance. However the depth of their responses can also include being a victim or a perpetrator of harsh violence. Blue unlike some other miasms, tends to perpetrate or receive their violence within the confines of their own four walls, outsiders being none the wiser. Purple with its suspicion and blaming nature imbibed by the red is the other miasm where such premeditated cruelty exists. Green is less likely to be a part of such venom because of their yellow influence. Red wants revenge, blue has trouble letting anything out so both of these miasms can make the worst of enemies. Brown by contrast will often take it all on board but remain nice all the same seemingly enduring the impossible for years on end. Green has their fair share of hatred and rage but this is often modified by the yellow need to drop things and move on with their lives. In this respect green will often need to move away or change their environment before forgiveness is possible.

Blue may keep everything hidden; often whilst presenting a smiling exterior. They have the ability to keep soldiering on as they have great inner strength and reserves but when they collapse will often take longer to recover and will experience a deeper response than the other miasms.

DEATH AND SALVATION

Death can be a major area of preoccupation for blue. Whether in the form of morbid dread or fascination, death is a presenting energy. They may have a belief they will die young or soon or it may be a serious dedication of study towards either proving or disproving the paranormal. In the same vein blue also has the strongest suicidal tendencies of all the miasms and can devote much of their time thinking and preparing for death. Another avenue of perusal can be seen in their continuous involvement and scrutiny of religion and mysticism, trying to find a meaning and a purpose for existence. Some may say this comes from an inherent sense of worthlessness hence some reason to exist must be sought, others suggest that the depth given by the miasm combined with its propensity for introspection means that grander topics of thought such as the meaning of life are inevitable. Only green can match the blue in their inquiring nature about the soul. Either way blue can seem obsessed with the notion of an afterlife and continual survival or perhaps as one patient suggested final and total release by obliteration. Turning to religion some from this miasmatic group may feel they are not worthy of salvation, doomed to eternal nothingness. I have seen some drawn towards religions that offer redemption, perhaps a hope given by a religion can counteract some of the hopelessness felt in their earthly life? Some may join a type of 'turn or burn' religion, a fundamentalist church that can show you how to be happy, to do what's right and to win favour. Some from this miasmatic family seem to need the black and white, the right or wrong and saved or damned rules these religions offer. Seemingly unable to believe in a God that can use personal judgment, many are drawn to religions that "know the answer" of how to prepare for their upcoming transfiguration. Whilst there is nothing fundamentally wrong with such beliefs they do with their emphasis on right and wrong tend to focus on the war waged between God and the Devil, and this concentration on the devil is the last thing some of the susceptible from this miasm need, nurturing the paranoia of evil and the devil can create great fear in some who may already have an instinctual fear of evil. Not all blue's fall into this category of course, and many get involved with many deep spiritual forms. Not concerned so much with an afterlife it becomes the preoccupation of some to try and avoid fear and suffering as best they can. Having already suffered enough, more torment would be like the straw that broke the camel's back, hence being filled to the brim they may have a strong fear of disease or anything else that may cause misery.

In the clinic blue patients have either near death accidents or near death experiences more often than patients from other miasms.

MIND; DOUBTFUL; souls welfare, of.

RELIGIOUS affections; spiritual improvement, desires.

DEPRESSION AND HAPPINESS

The pursuit of happiness and its counter energy depression is probably the single most dominating feature of this miasm. Many blue patients present as being light and laugh more often than patients from other miasms. They are cheerful about everything and don't want to discuss painful aspects of their current or past life. Most are able to brush off difficulties and appear not to be affected by the memory of past hurts. But this is only an image they portray and blue will hurt just as deeply as anyone else.

MIND; CHEERFULNESS, gaiety, happiness; tendency.

MIND; LAUGHING; tendency.

Once contentment cannot be found and life offers little in the way of enjoyment, they may withdraw from life into a shell of a world, resigned to the continuum of indifference and nothingness. If they can bond with someone they may invest all their happiness into one person family or love, which is fine providing it lasts however if it breaks apart they may have nothing else in their lives in which to live for. The same may occur in a business. While it is progressing there is always something to do, their mind can be diverted into other avenues, saving them from the perpetual boredom and bleakness that awaits them when alone.

There can be a tendency towards suicide but this is not the note leaving or revengeful type of suicide, using death to cause even more pain to those around them. Suicide for blue is often just a release from pain a slipping into nothingness that frees one of suffering and despair too strong to overcome they find release in any form they can.

Sometimes the depression that consumes them causes no pain at all, as they are too indifferent to life to remember what happiness was. Nothing exists except this single moment and this moment doesn't bear thinking about even if they could. There is a void, a nothingness that cannot be filled even if they knew how. Not taking anything in, not responding to life or feeling, not wanting, not experiencing, not knowing – this is the depression of blue.

Physically this energy loss can manifest as a depleted and depressed immune system, causing continuous repeating infections. Some of these conditions although annoying are relatively harmless, such as always suffering from a cold, sinus problems or a lack of energy, while other symptoms can be more chronic and serious in their nature. The nature of this miasm in disease is to infiltrate and destroy and it is given free rein to do so by an immune system that offers a yielding resistance. In fact this type of resistance and conceding ground can be a miasmatic theme of blue.

At this point it is important to remember that miasmatic themes are not full time issues. Take the depression of blue for instance; although deep and miserable, it makes only a small proportion of their life if at all. Someone can still belong to this miasm and suffer from depression, the only expression of this miasm they may exhibit. But the depression may in the grand scheme of things take up a small proportion of their time, being relatively happy and stable for ninety five percent of their life and depressed for the other five means that apart from these periods of blue exacerbation they are perfectly functional in every other way. Like somebody with a bad back, it may only cause real problems every now and then however the sufferer is always constantly aware of its existence and lives in fear of its reoccurrence, but in times when their back is not playing up they live perfectly normally.

MIND; LAUGHING; tendency; never.

MIND; SMILING; never.

MIND; SADNESS, despondency, depression, melancholy; aversion to see her children from sadness; children to whom he is devotedly attached become burdensome.

MIND; ENNUI, boredom mental.

MIND; INDIFFERENCE, apathy; dead, everything seems to him, nothing makes a vivid impression upon his mind.

MIND; MORAL affections; antisocial.

MIND; WEARY of life.

MIND; INDIFFERENCE, apathy; business affairs.

INSANITY AND MENTAL INSTABILITY

'All this promiscuity and philandering didn't make the nobility any happier or healthier. Frances I of France was as cavalier as any courtier until syphilis sprang three leaks in his bladder. King Henry the VIII of England and his syphilitic exploits condemned the Tudor line to extinction. Ivan the terrible of Russia lived up to his name by boiling, burning, flogging and skewering his enemies in great numbers. Treponema finally ended his insanity with a brain seizure during a game of chess.'

Syphilis as a disease exemplifies the extent to which this miasm can reach. By understanding the stages of the disease, we can understand the potential of the miasm. This being the case consider the following: *'Within two hundred years of its arrival, it became the 'great imitator" and harder to diagnose. Adapting to long life, the treponema signalled its youth with chancres and swollen lymph glands, middle age with joint pains and hoarse throats and old age with heart attacks and insanity. After fifty years of coexistence with the disease, many syphilitics also went blind or started to walk like a drunk with a broken foot.'*

It is no surprise then that brain disease is a prime pathological indicator for this miasm. Whether in the form of eccentricity or a classified and labelled medical condition such as Alzheimer's disease or mental retardation both bear the characteristic hallmark of the presence of blue. Varying in degree, blue may range from a recoverable nervous breakdown, to severe mental degeneration and imbecility.

The brain, special senses and the bones bear the brunt of the blue stigma. One of the physiological pathologies contributing to this blue feeling of madness is their persistent and continual insomnia. Driving them literally mad with frustration and tiredness it is no wonder blue dreads the night.

Blue can turn to drugs and alcohol as a means of coping with or escaping from the enemy in their heads. All miasms have some part of themselves that seems to turn against them as that particular area bears the brunt of their miasmatic disease. The reproductive system and musculature in red, the kidneys, lungs or nervous systems of green, the digestive system in yellow and for blue it is the bones and the brain. Understanding Hering's law it is easy to see how deep this miasmatic impact is.

A mental or physical degeneration of the brain may disallow in some any relief or respite as your brain is with you where ever you go the illness for some is all pervading and inescapable. During the night when nearly all external stimuli ceases, the blue mind can come to life, perhaps constructively being at their most creative or doing their best work, perhaps even taking on night work knowing these hours would suit them better. At its worst, the night can be a torment of rushing thoughts and sleeplessness.

INSANITY, madness.

MIND; HOWLING.

MIND; ESCAPE, attempts to; run away, to.

ADDICTIONS AND OBSESSIONAL BEHAVIOUR

Obsessive tendencies can display themselves in various forms; gambling, sex, substance abuse, rituals, cleaning, work, the range is endless.

Without doubt the most common of all their obsessions is in reference to their health. In a more positive display, they can be health fanatics, devoting their whole life to different regimens, diets and vitamins. Becoming super fit, their lives may be ruled by an exercise routine around which all other aspects of life come second. It does not have to be competitive nor are they necessarily trying to reach a particular goal, it is just another expression of how the miasm can exhibit its obsessive compulsive tendencies.

In a more negative form their preoccupation with health can turn to hypochondria. The patient especially fears fatal diseases like cancer or AIDS, often greatly out of proportion to his state of health, age or family history.

The array in which an obsession with health can exhibit itself can be extensive ranging from health care to hypochondria to a morbid fear of germs and accidents. Making their house fool proof and impossible for an accident to occur is as strong a display, as continuous cleaning with every anti bacterial potion on the market.

Work is another prime outlet for this type of behaviour. Most strongly represented in remedies like Aurum, it may be seen as a dedication to hard work, or committed to being a good provider, always the first to arrive and the last to leave, oftentimes working through weekends and deep into the night. Rewarded and applauded by the company it often hides the true obsessional nature of the person behind it.

Blue need to know the guidelines and to understand the rules. They will check on how things are to be done and confirm and reconfirm in an obsessive way. This is their attempt to keep control in their lives and to keep the unknown from their door. In some cases disguised as a need to "know more" once it is understood the patient is blue this type of behaviour will make more sense.

MIND; SATYRIASIS (Nymphomania).

MALE; COITION; enjoyment; extreme.

FEMALE; COITION; enjoyment; extreme.

MIND; DELUSIONS, imaginations; dirt, dirty; he is.

MIND; FEAR; disease, of; impending; contagious, epidemic, infection.

MIND; WASHING; always; hands.

DRUGS AND ALCOHOL

The more yielding nature of blue means that they are susceptible to the impact of both drugs and alcohol. This is also seen in green, brown and purple all known for having remedies under the rubric alcoholism. However the opposite can also be true and blue can be a teetotaler or never touch drugs in an attempt to remain healthy and pure.

It has often been speculated that alcoholism and drug addiction may be genetic, but without an understanding of the miasms, geneticists may forever be debating this question. There is no doubt that blue have genetically acquired a susceptibility to easy alcohol addiction however this does not mean that they will never be able to control alcohol as there must also be the addition of other co-factors to create the addiction.

Magic and rituals may be another area where blue shows itself, believing in hexes and talismans to ward off evil. This can take the form of praying and crossing constantly or it can so superstitious that their whole lives are ruined by fear and paranoia. Never allowing themselves to relax they can continuously occupy their time with séances, ouija boards and charms.

Ritualistic behaviour may transcend into physical manifestations rather than just behavioural traits. Constant rocking or the twirling of their thumbs, excessive repeated blinking or winking can be amongst the most common observable signs.

MIND; ALCOHOLISM, dipsomania; hereditary.

FAMILY AND FRIENDS

The family plays a pivotal role in the life of blue. In its most positive form this will mean that blue make caring and loving parents even if the emotional connection may appear to be lighter. However in some it may take on a less than positive form. Some can have an aversion to one or other members of their family. This can be demonstrated by rebelliousness to a particular person. To bickering and inhouse fighting leading to mistrust or indifference towards the other members of the house. Not limited to the childhood home, it may extend itself into the marital home again manifesting as indifference or a desire to dissolve and run away from the whole arrangement. For those that have the ability to project their inner turmoil onto an outside personality, thing or group; the family is most often the brunt of all of their considerable pent up aggression and distress, blaming them for the way they feel about themselves. There might be real validity behind this thought in the form of abuse as blue can have cruelty around them or it may be projection.

MIND; ABUSIVE, insulting; family and children, to.

MIND; DELUSIONS, imaginations; marriage, must dissolve.

MIND; ESCAPE, attempts to; run away, to.

CHILDISHNESS AND NAIVITY

In contrast to depression and indifference is their capacity for sensitivity combined with a lightness which may appear as either childishness or naivety. Making jokes, laughing and seeing the lighter side of life is the counter energy to depth and depression. Often fun to be around, blue can have many friends and be part of large groups. When carried too far they can seem to be frivolous and even wasteful.

MIND; FRIVOLOUS.

MIND; SQUANDERS.

Being prone to introspection makes blue sensitive and perceptive, it can create a depth of understanding unavailable to many other miasms. It is the blue that makes green so sensitive to thunderstorms and propels them towards beauty and harmonious environments, and it is the blue that gives the brown their reputation for keeping the peace.

It portrays calm acceptance. 'A quietness of spirit that presents integrity'. Because they are internal, blue understands that happiness is in the way you look at things. For this reason they may be the most honest and trustworthy as they are often the only miasm that doesn't want anything from you. Understanding depression can help many to achieve enjoyment in the little things. They can appreciate that happiness comes from a state not a possession. Knowing what its like to suffer helps in the pleasure of the day to day, some may see it as a little life, not aspiring to anything others may see it for what it really is; a contentment and existence in the moment.

SPECIAL SENSES AND SENSITIVITY

One thing about blue that separates them from the other miasms is their lack of want. Indeed most crave very little in the way of 'things', just the basics and a roof over their head, a happy family and food on the table. Perhaps this is the positive side of indifference, often interpreted as an indifference to people it may also mean an indifference to the glitter and show of modern life. Described by some as quiet or antisocial they will care very little for the razzamatazz preferring instead to withdraw to a quieter more simple life. Being unable to offer any great resistance to outside pressures, their instinctive reaction is to withdraw trying to find calm and tranquillity within their lives, they crave an 'orderly environment free from upsets and disturbance'.

Like orange, blue understands deep emotional pain and having experienced it will do anything to stop its reoccurrence. Therefore they strive to achieve harmony both in their relationships and their environment. Pain may bring understanding, and as a consequence blue can have a clarity that other miasms may lack. If unable to achieve this quiescence, depression, heart problems or addictions may ensue. Chaos being the enemy of serenity, they may attempt to control everything or being a miasm of extremes, may decide to relinquish in order to keep the peace. Remember, yellow is trying to eradicate and overcome, red is attempting to contain but blue is giving ground. Therefore conciliation should be one of their strongest points, provided they don't concede too much. The other side of the coin is a hard and unforgiving nature. Using miasmatic themes in broad contexts can sometimes be helpful in understanding how different themes emerge. If we take the two major complexes of blue, green and purple and apply broad themes, we begin to see the miasmatic differences between each group. For example blue is conciliation and giving ground, whereas yellow is overcoming and profiting, therefore green will concede a little to gain more in the long run. Red is containment and control, therefore in purple to give ground is to lose control or seen another way, purple could see conciliation as an embarrassing loss of face, prepared to accept nothing rather than a little.

Blue affects all the special senses and the organs that are responsible for them. The nose, the eyes and the mouth are all both structurally and functionally disturbed and eroded. Metaphorically this means that the way they view events will be more unique than any other group. They may have a distorted way of viewing the world, as input is limited or deranged. They cannot and do not experience life in the same way as the other miasms. This means that there will be some who live on an entirely different earth than the rest of us. With either their special senses on overload or hardly working at all means even a little bit of stimulus can be too much. This can manifest as a physical incapability to interpret stimuli as found in mental retardation making it impossible to fully perceive the vastness and intricacies of the world, or it may come from an overload that makes any new input too much to handle. This being the case they may try and shrink their world down to a more manageable size. This to some degree is what an obsession is, a total focus on one thing as that one thing is comprehendible. Continuous repetition is another example of a shrinking, more understandable and less threatening world.

Brown is a miasm also known for its compulsive behaviour, while green is a miasm known for its obsessiveness towards a particular topic, project or work of art. Both of these miasms get this trait from blue. The difference between green and blue for example is that because of the yellow, their obsession must have some constructive and productive purpose. With brown we can sometimes see the combination of the ambition of yellow combined with the wild confusion of red and the obsessiveness of blue. A remedy exemplifying these three is Arsenicum. They need to be productive and get things done (yellow) but unlike green it's not in one particular area as they have the confusion of red. Trying obsessively to place this confusion into some kind of order so they can be productive makes them generally fastidious (brown) rather than just conscientious about their work (green).

BLUE CASES

CASE 1 – Ms J S aged thirty-two

Ms J S came into the clinic complaining of severe aching in her bones. Her left leg was swollen and she felt both numbness and hot pain particularly after motion. Tests show her bones are deteriorating and on two occasions she has suffered bad breaks for no apparent reason. Her white cell count is abnormal and she fears she will get cancer. There is a history of TB, diabetes, cancer and syphilis in her family. Her appetite is low and she dislikes meat. Every year she gets at least three major colds or flus. She was violently raped at twenty two and this led to a pregnancy that ended in a miscarriage just prior to a planned abortion. During the rape she was stabbed in the thigh. Her father was abusive to her and her siblings all through their childhood. Both parents are holocaust survivors and she has become very interested in this heritage. She is writing a book about their experiences. She hasn't told her father about this as she finds it hard to face him. Her relationship consists of one major and two minor relationships – all three men were abusive to her, one tried to kill her in a drunken temper. She lives on her own and has no further interest in a relationship – she doesn't want to have children as she does not want to pass on her "bad genes". She is suspicious of men's motives and would rather be alone. When she is tired she often sees spirits or faces in front of her. She is nervous and can't bear noise. This sensitivity makes sleep difficult and sometimes she stays up all night.

This patient first came to me in 1996 and was prescribed Carcinosin which had no result. Later she was given Staphysagria but again no result. During the first two consultations no miasmatic prescription was applied as the theory was still in its embryonic stage. Later as the theory developed and became more practical, Ms S, because of her many blue features, became one of the first test cases, with stunning results.

The rubrics chosen for her case were

MIND; SUSPICIOUSNESS, mistrustfulness.

GENERALITIES; NIGHT, nine p.m. – five a.m.; agg.

GENERALITIES; FOOD and drinks; meat; aversion.

GENERALITIES; BONES, complaints of.

GENERALITIES; COLD; tendency to take, taking cold agg.

MIND; DELUSIONS, imaginations; faces, sees.

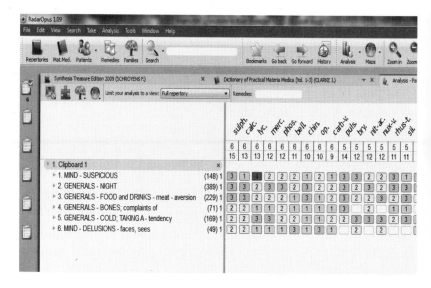

Facial features

Red

Nose ball shaped end

Lips full

Eyes protrude

Blue

Hairline very high

Forehead curved

Strong alae nasi lines

Large ears

Asymmetrical - eyes and nose

Eyes upturned

Vertical lines cheeks

Pointed chin

The only blue remedy in the repertorisation was Mercury. On questioning it was discovered she also sweated profusely on exertion. Using her as a test case Mercury 30 was given daily until improvement. One month later she was feeling wonderful and not nearly as fearful about getting cancer. The remedy was stopped. She started sleeping and felt relaxed. She was taking a holiday to the United States to further her book research, so couldn't see me for the next appointment, but on her return rang to say she was still feeling well. She had met a man with whom she planned to live and her bone pain was better. Her next round of tests showed a dramatic improvement in bone density.

CASE 1 – Ms T L aged twenty-two

Ms T L presents with eczema and stress symptoms. She is an engineering student and the pressure of impending exams is difficult for her. Her mother had previously contacted me concerned about the degree to which she will study as she forgets to eat and drink unless meals are placed in front of her and she is made to stop. Sometimes she will not leave her room for two days. It is as if the rest of the world is forgotten. The eczema has developed slowly over the last eighteen months and is copper coloured and concentrated in both armpits, the legs and around the genitals. Many natural substances have been tried without result. Further discussion around her study habits revealed that when she concentrates she unknowingly pulls the hair from her arms, legs and head. She is later surprised to find blood on her arms, legs and face.

The rubrics chosen for her case were

MIND; MUTILATE his body, inclination to.

MIND; AVERSION; society.

MIND; COMPULSIVE disorders.

SKIN; ERUPTIONS; coppery.

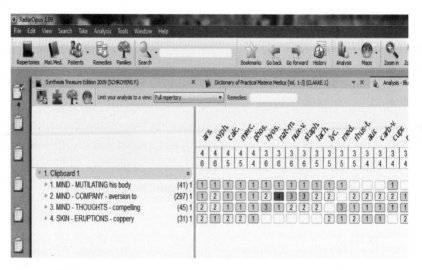

Facial features

Yellow

Thin lips

Red

Straight hairline

Blue

High hairline

Forehead curved

Eyes deep set

Asymmetry – eyes, nose

Crooked sharp teeth

Ms T L displays classic destructive blue tendencies and her facial features also show the dominance of blue. Syphilinum 1M single dose resulted in a complete clearing of the eczema and a less obsessive attitude towards studying. She no longer pulls the hair from her body. No further dose was required. Three months later on seeing her mother as a patient she reports that her daughter is still doing well.

THE GENERALS OF BLUE

SENSATIONS

Violent pains

Cold pains

Buzzing sensations

Vibrating sensations

Knotted sensations

Crushing sensations

Tremors

FOOD

Aversion to all food

Aversion to meat

Aggravation from meat

Desires coffee

Desires alcohol

Aggravation from alcohol

Aggravation from sweets and sugar

AGGRAVATIONS

Night

During sleep

Wet weather

Cold and warm weather

Sitting

Bandaging/wraps

AMELIORATIONS

Light

Sunshine

Walking

Motion

Cool weather

PATHOLOGY

Brain. Bones. Atrophy of the glands. Vicarious menstruation. Genital warts. **Fissures**. Optical nerve. **Special senses. Green/yellow discharges. Heart. Ulceration. Linear**/transverse pain. Sweating. Falling of hair, teeth and nails. Necrosis and **destruction** of tissue. Orifices. Scarlet fever. Glands.

CHAPTER 17

Miasmatic Themes - Syco-Psora (Orange)

INAPPROPRIATE RELATIONSHIPS

Driven by an insatiable need to be loved, orange may instinctively turn their attention to the "strays" of the pack. In the same way as a child adopts an abandoned kitten, many see themselves as a saviour, rescuing the needy and misunderstood, who will, in turn, be forever grateful, a loyal companion who will love them and support them and follow them to the ends of the earth. This is orange naivety at its worst and it often sets in motion a train of events that end, predictably, in tragedy.

This is the most emotional and needy miasm, often containing an energy of grief, deception and cruelty. Remedies like Nat Mur. and Ignatia are well known for their predisposition to fall in love with unobtainable or inappropriate people. In past repertories, "inappropriate" meant falling in love with someone married, but inappropriate may also mean falling in love with a person completely incompatible or unsuitable to their wellbeing. Some find themselves in predicaments where their romantic hopes are dashed, replaced with grief and despair, and to add insult to injury, because their energy hasn't changed, some will leave their partner only to fall in love with another person of exactly the same ilk.

Often attracted to those that will do them the most harm, some are drawn towards needy or addictive types that require a carer, more than a lover. Nat Mur. is a prime example of a martyr ready to take on the responsibility of saviour. As a practitioner to orange you will hear stories of deception, infidelity and repeated naivety, often stemming from the belief they can mould, reshape and change their project/lover. In some cases it may be true, but most times this idealism will lead to delusion and grief.

The other side of the coin is they can be the emotionally overburdening and needy one. Placing high demands upon their partner and those around them while at the same time being intolerant of any pressures or expectations placed on them, some from this miasm can be so desperate for attention they become emotionally selfish and unrealistic. They require saving rather than being a saviour.

Deception and the ailments from it, are one of the keys to understanding the energy of this miasm. Not always the one who will be deceived, orange is capable of being the deceiver, often being susceptible to the charms of another.

Some find themselves loving the person others love to hate. This new partner may be socially unacceptable or disliked. In hindsight I have heard some confess their relationship was formed more out of spite or to show their liberal thinking, than out of actual love.

Sometimes these "underdogs" have deep-seated and habitual problems; violence, addictions, self-centredness and abuse; it is not surprising to find some of these orange saviours becoming targets.

MIND; AILMENTS from; love; disappointed, unhappy.

MIND; LOVE; married man or coachman, with.

MIND; LOVE; falling in love easily.

JEALOUSY, DECEPTION AND SHAME

Being a slave to their emotions, orange find they fall in and out of love easily and consistently. However most are neither flirtatious nor lascivious, they simply get swept up in the romance or the perceived romance. Sometimes they read far more into a look than they should, prone to misinterpretations, they continually set themselves up for emotional injuries.

Many have a strong moral code and can be quite conservative hence their infatuations come to no physical end and remain a love from afar. This is the romantic idealism and unrequited love made famous by Ignatia and Nat Mur. Swept up in their emotions, an affair may take place so rapidly that they may feel they haven't had time to breathe let alone time to think. Against their moral code, some will find it difficult to comprehend it is *they* who are doing the deceiving.

Orange has a tendency to fall in love with those they see frequently, constantly projecting their desperation for the dream onto someone around them then regretting this projection, they feel embarrassed and guilty about their fantasies, and avoid the person in question or treat them indifferently. All the while the brunt of the fantasy remains unaware of the emotional ebbs and flows going on around them. If an affair does occur despite the heartfelt love they may feel for their new partner, many will not get past the guilt and shame of their actions. Whilst they may move on and have a happy and productive life in their new relationship, it should not be surprising to find most of their pathological aetiology having its origin from this point. Consciously they may have progressed but scratch the surface and you will see they are still caught in the energy of shame and guilt.

MIND; GRIEF; deception, from.

MIND; AILMENTS from; excitement; general symptoms from.

MIND; IDEALISTIC.

MIND; ANXIETY; conscience.

ONCE THE ROMANCE IS OVER

"Deceived" by their miasm, those drawn to the underdog now find they must live with their mistake. Orange is a romantic idealist and, as such, many are demanding of their partners. For their partner, to be picked up out of the emotional gutter is one thing, to have to pay back the favour is quite another. Often the partner of orange does not feel the same obligation that orange believe they owe. Seeing it from the partner's point of view, orange took on the role of saviour, benefactor and lover, they began with this role and it should continue – this is what the relationship is based on. Picking someone up and putting them back on their feet, orange can be heartbroken when they exercise their newfound mobility and leave. From the orange point of view, they were attempting to help someone help themselves. They did not sign up for continuous nurturing.

Unfortunately some have chosen a partner not deserving of their respect. Orange cannot love somebody they cannot respect and they will not have sex with someone they don't love. Aversion to coition is a rubric that runs through many orange remedies. Like yellow that has embarrassment over sexual issues, orange may find themselves in the same position of either "aversion to coition" or "ailments from coition" because they cannot be intimate physically with someone whom they are not intimate with romantically. Once respect for their partner is lost, there may be moments of closeness but general intimacy will vanish.

FEMALE; COITION; aversion to.

FEMALE; COITION; enjoyment; absent.

CHEATING

Always ready to give people the benefit of the doubt, many find themselves in a position of being exploited and manipulated. They want to trust, and they need to believe, even though their head is alerting them to facts that simply do not add up, their heart will over ride their gut instinct refusing to believe the obvious. To outsiders they can seem naïve, a sucker being taken for a ride and refusing to accept the evident by finding comfort in the lie. The amount of times the topic of infidelity or deception will arise during a consultation from someone from this miasm is disproportionate, showing it as a central theme.

Even though grief is a miasmatic theme of the orange group, people belonging to this group will still respond differently. One person may become catatonic (Nat Mur.) another hysterical (Ignatia) or aggressive (Nux Vomica). This is why an array of medicines exists within each miasmatic group.

GUILT AND TRAGEDY

A sense that they have neglected to do their duty or feelings of guilt are strong character aspects. So far we have discussed their justifiable guilt, but for many from this miasmatic group a sense of guilt or neglect is unjustifiable. This emotion can be stifling, making some excessively conservative. Some may gain a reputation for stability, never risking or doing anything wrong or inappropriate for it would make them feel guilty to the point they could not live with themselves. This "righteousness" can consume their energy as they take on the burden of increasing responsibility, performing every task to guarantee that the job is done properly. Becoming intolerant of others they can have a short temper being over stressed and tired. They need help but they do not trust the help that is being offered.

MIND; DELUSIONS, imaginations; crime; committed, he had.

MIND; DELUSIONS, imaginations; neglected; duty, his.

MIND; REJECTS everything offered to him.

LOSS

An energy of loss, grief and death can surround orange hence why so many remedies belonging to it are known for grief and trauma, Ignatia, Nat Mur. and Nux Vomica being just a few. This miasm should be suspected when a patient tells a story of one tragedy after another – here it will resemble blue very closely.

Whilst in their day-to-day life, they may be stoic keeping up a brave face to those around them, their sleep and dreams tell a different story. Horrible and sad dreams, dreams of death and calamity, all can be experienced constantly. They may fight all their battles in their dreams such as in Ferrum Met. They are easily upset by music, as music is an emotional trigger that brings to the fore everything they are trying to suppress.

Rejecting things asked for is a strong symptom of Chamomilla and highlights another character trait present in many of the remedies that belong to this miasm. Literally this rubric is used to show the capricious nature of the person needing Chamomilla, but it can also be extended to more lateral concepts particularly in reference to their need for help and support and its subsequent refusal as just discussed.

Being the most emotionally demonstrative of all the miasms, grief or distress cause pain that is almost intolerable. Remedies like Chamomilla, Coffea and Ignatia help serve to highlight how quickly orange can be driven to hysteria. Demanding sympathy from those around them rather than having it given willingly, they are far less likely to get the reassurance and emotional support they desperately need. Feeling let down and unsupported they become angry and resentful. Deciding to hide their emotions rather than be open with them, the brave face can become such a way of life they may be considered cold or aloof. Many are hysterical by nature, even though self-educated to be contained. The miasm can still be seen by the mayhem that surrounds them. Here they differ from red in that red are often more contained and controlling, keeping secrets and motives hidden from the view of others, but with orange, hysteria reigns and as such tension and calamity, lies and deception are never far behind. To some, life is a continual soap opera of drama, despair and volatility.

MIND; CONSOLATION; agg.

MIND AILMENTS from; death; parents or friends, of.

MIND; DREAMS; battles.

MIND; MUSIC; agg.

MIND; MUSIC; aversion to.

MIND; HYSTERIA.

SYMPATHY AND CHARITY

Dreams and internalised grief are common ways their over exuberant emotions display themselves. Some will turn the anger they feel into zeal in an attempt to harness their sense of anger and injustice. Being so emotional this miasmatic group has a sympathetic nature towards the suffering of others.

Not all sympathy comes from personal experience. Many have a strong sense of compassion not born from pain. Some have a natural instinct to help. They may become embroiled in a fight for justice, defending the downtrodden, again surrounding themselves with the energy of the suffering, and the needy. They are a fighter looking for a fight, a knight looking for a damsel in distress, but if providence does not provide a damsel, then orange will go out of their way to find one. What they are fighting may not be as important as having something to fight for.

Sometimes the emotional demands of others can draw them consistently outside of their home. Having to continually attend to emergencies and calamities, many spend more time on their 'cases' than they do with their partners and children. It is their family that now feels bereft, misunderstood and deserted. Their family may feel they have no one to turn to in *their* time of need, it may even cause the breakdown of their relationship, fulfilling the energetic pattern that dominates them. Whether they help the emotionally needy or they are the emotionally needy is irrelevant, either expression is merely orange exerting its influence. However, brown supersedes all other miasms in their adoption of a cause.

MIND; AILMENTS from; cares, worries.

MIND; INJUSTICE, cannot support.

MIND; SYMPATHETIC, compassionate.

HYSTERIA, QUARRELS AND CHAOS

Orange, like red, is hurried and impetuous; as a consequence they may be scattered, disorganised, hysterical and frenzied. Their world can be chaotic. Displaying their emotions makes them impulsive and obvious. But sometimes social interaction calls for subtlety not blatancy, and as a consequence some are misjudged or may cause friction. Demonstrative shows of affection towards somebody outside of their own relationship may be nothing but friendly expressions to orange, but it may be regarded as invasive and flirtatious by others. Arguments can arise, orange may find themselves embroiled in a situation of conflict. Touchy-feely behaviour is most often given by people in love/lust with one another. Being touchy-feely people by nature, others may believe there is more than just friendship in their touch, orange can forget or fail to understand that this behaviour is, by some, exclusively reserved for the intimate.

Due to their internal emotional chaos and instability, many seek their shadow side by choosing partners who are stable, linear and self contained. Whilst orange may be secure and stable in this relationship, they may also find their partners so stable that they lack the ability for emotional demonstration leaving them unfulfilled and their love unrequited. Being half yellow, orange has a practical side and may offset their red yearning for closeness by a shared project or business. The combination of yellow (embarrassment) and red (containment) means orange can be "cold" and undemonstrative often accused of being too safe or frigid, remaining uncommitted and uninvolved so they can shield themselves from any outside stimulus. They are unwilling to take part and insulate themselves from direct participation by dealing with what they must mechanically and artificially. Homoeopathy is used to understanding energy as both sided of a coin. What is true of a theme must also be true for its opposite. While many may be emotionally hysterical and needy there will be just as many who are undemonstrative and overly rational.

MIND; AFFECTIONATE.

BUSINESS

Orange have an inherent belief they are right. They are missionaries as well as campaigners. In order to "save", one must come from a position of authority. Another expression of their conservative nature is their righteousness. This brings them into conflict with those around them as things must be done their way. To others, they may seem dictatorial and volatile such as the Nux Vomica temperament. Their drive for efficiency and their need to be right make them intolerant of mistakes. Many prefer to be the boss rather than the subordinate. Their rightness and natural leaning towards efficiency means they are far more comfortable giving orders than taking them.

Righteousness also implies a strict moral code and practical conservatism. These more conservative types are shining examples of the "protestant work ethic", highly moral, extremely driven, self contained with temperance. This is in complete contrast to the more hysterical types. Anger and frustration are being turned to enthusiasm and fervour.

Orange are "right" and as a natural consequence everything they do must be right. They enjoy efficiency for its own sake. How things are done is as important as what is trying to be achieved. They can be at war against the sloppy and inadequate, intolerant of compromise as compromise is seen as giving ground and this is not the orange way. They are uncompromising; others must raise their standards rather than orange lowering theirs. Uncompromising is as strong a central theme as deception, grief, hysteria, it is still another way of being demanding.

They are employees that never leave until the job is completed. They take work home, they get in early, they leave late, they do not relax, they keep thinking about a problem until a solution is found, they are efficient, they are driven, they take on more and more responsibility, they mistrust others' abilities – they lose sleep, they are angry, they are short-tempered, they are stressed – orange is a nervous breakdown waiting to happen.

Loyalty is a major part of their character, in the workplace it displays itself clearly, they will be rock solid in their support of their superiors and the work expectations of the company.

Seriousness is another keyword for orange. They take their romances seriously, their work seriously and their roles seriously. Indeed sometimes it can be an uphill battle to get any fun out of them at all. It's not that they don't want to have fun, it's just that they have become so used to their self-imposed containment they have forgotten how to let go and relax, hence they become tense and inhibited.

One of their major physiological complaints is cramps and spasms as too is high blood pressure, sleeplessness and restless agitation. When we begin to understand what drives the orange miasm, their symptoms become self-explanatory. They have an inability to relax. They are restless and busy, always looking for something to do. There is a saying that if you want something done – give it to a busy person. Unable to say no, they take on more tasks than they are capable of performing, soon becoming overstressed and unbearable to live with. They may turn to stimulants to aid them in the extra energy they need to get through their workload, beginning to overload their systems they risk the possibility of a complete nervous breakdown. Whilst most other miasms have a fear of some illness or disease such as cancer or heart disease, it is interesting to note that this is the only miasm that has a fear of getting a stomach ulcer.

MIND; Always in the right.

MIND; AILMENTS from; discords between; chief and subordinates.

MIND; CONSCIENTIOUS about trifles.

MIND; RESPONSIBILITY. MIND; FEAR; stomach ulcer, of.

ORANGE CASES

CASE 1 Mr E aged forty-seven

Mr E aged forty seven presented with breathing difficulties including sleep apnoea. He can never breathe out of both nostrils at the same time and often wakes choking. He has had a cough for the last six months after a cold – the cough is a dry tickle which is < talking, < night, < cold air.

Other problems include dizzy spells where he feels as if he will fall over and faint. He has fainted a couple of times. This fainting feeling and his breathlessness are worse ascending.

Light-headedness that lasts for a time then leaves. He suffers with colds on a regular basis often every two weeks.

Mr E is overweight and has tried all sorts of dieting regimens as well as exercise programs but to no avail. His wife, who is also at the consultation, points out her concern at how little he actually eats – she believes that he cannot drop his intake any lower than it already is.

History of dizzy spells near collapse – he becomes light headed and clammy.

Regular episodes of chest pain which have been described as stabbing and "extreme pressure". He feels this pain continually both day and night.

In his personality Mr E describes himself as efficient and driven and extremely short tempered. He is a production manager for a large and continuously growing company and has a lot of responsibility both in terms of deadlines, product and staff management. He describes his job as "a high pressure" occupation. He takes great pride in his work and values his contribution to the company. He is the first to admit that he gets "very worked up" when things don't run to schedule. He becomes frustrated and irritable and the whole floor will know his mood. He states that he has done various forms of stress relief so he is not as tough as he used to be. In the past he described himself as "a very hard task master". He gets in to work early and comes home late. He describes his managerial character as "fair, but firm". He walks in his spare time and does french polishing and cabinet making as a hobby and as a way to relax his mind. When questioned on how effective a relaxation tool the cabinet making is – his reply was to laugh and state "not very."

Q. Where does your mind naturally go to once your tasks are finished and you have some spare time?

A. I don't have any spare time. If I do I will only worry about what is going on at work while I'm not there. The plant runs twenty four hours a day – I'm only there for twelve of them. I need to do other things otherwise I'll find myself on the phone checking up on everyone.

Q. Do you have any hobbies?

A. A few years ago my blood pressure was sky high. I knew I had to take up something to try and relax me. I walk around a lot at work, but I decided to take up walking as an exercise after work as well. In the end though I had to take up something else as I would just think about work while I walked.

Q. Have you found anything that can take your mind off work?

A. I like working with my hands. I need to be busy all the time. If I'm not busy with my hands I'm busy with my mind. I took up cabinet making because it involves skill and high concentration. While doing this I can find that I forget about work because I'm concentrating so intensely on whatever project I have chosen to make.

Q. Does this help relieve your stress?

At this point both Mr E and his wife begin to laugh.

A. No in fact I think it has added to the stress. It's true I don't think about work when I'm cabinet making but the slightest thing that goes wrong and I'm in a furious rage. Many times bits of wood have gone flying around my shed with swear words not far behind.

Q. Why is it so stressful for you?

A. My abilities are not up to my expectations quite yet. I know how I want something to look but often I can't quite make it to the level that is in my mind's eye. This is infuriating – I hate doing things that don't work out the way I want them to.

Q. When are you at your worst?

A. When I'm driving to work. I leave before the traffic but coming home I'm right in the peak hour, but sitting in a car doing nothing sends my blood pressure sky high and my temper reaches boiling point. If anyone in the traffic does something stupid I feel like I could almost kill them.

The rubrics chosen for the case were:

CHEST; PAIN; pressing.

MIND; ANGER, irascibility; tendency; easily.

GENERALITIES; ASCENDING; agg.

GENERALITIES; FAINTNESS, fainting; tendency; morning.

GENERALITIES; COLD; tendency to take, taking cold agg.; abnormally easy.

RESPIRATION; ARRESTED.

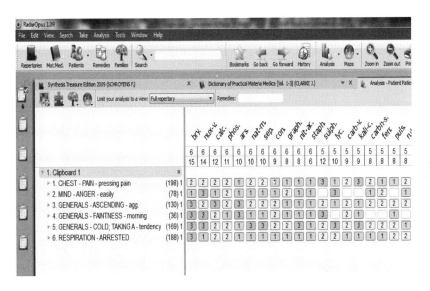

Facial features

Yellow

Eyes, close set

Prominent front teeth

Compact smile

Thin lips

Red

Gaps between the teeth

Full smile

Exopthalmic eyes

Wide nose

From the following list – Nux Vom., Ferr., and Nat Mur. are all orange remedies. This means that our selection must be made from this group. From this point standard homoeopathic skills are applied in relation to essence and keynotes and Nux Vom. was selected. Again this highlights that this new miasmatic method serves to refine accepted homoeopathic case taking and remedy selection.

Follow up – Nux Vom. 1M

Two weeks later Mr E reported that he wasn't worrying as much, his mood swings were not as bad and his stress levels were down. He has not had any dizzy spells. He has an itchy scalp late at night. The pain in his chest has lessened but is still continuous. He feels that he has another cold coming on. Mr E felt the medicine had been beneficial but he was slipping back. Nux Vom. 10M was prescribed. One month later he says he is 90 per cent better, most noticeably, when he is in the car he remains calm. He has been thirsty at night (a new symptom) and some mild stomach cramps – "not annoying just there" (a new symptom). The chest pain occurs only fleetingly but is no longer continuous nor painful. He had no dizzy spells and his breathing during sleep is better. Occasionally he will wake but not often. No remedy was given. Two months later Mr E describes himself as "stable" – he is going with the flow and his sleeping is fine. Sleep apnoea is fine – sleeping through and has had one or two dizzy spells but only minor. He has had a couple of heart pains under very stressful moments.* No remedy was given. One month later he is starting to become irritable again and work is getting him down. He is getting aggressive in the traffic and his chest pains have returned and have become more continuous. He has also experienced heart palpitations but his breathing and sleep are normal. Nux Vom. 10M was repeated. Two months later he continues to feels fine. He has had no colds and breathing is normal – no chest pain or dizzy spells.

*It is important to note that previous to coming to the clinic Mr E had had his heart checked on a number of occasions and there is no organic problem.

CASE 2 – T C aged ten

His presenting problem is migraines. These have occurred every ten to fourteen days for the last eighteen months driving him into bed often for two days. The pain is worse on the right side and he describes it as thumping. There are no apparent modalities.

Q. When did these first start?

A. [Mother] He had just come back from a weekend with his father and was dropped off early complaining of feeling unwell. By that evening he had a migraine.

Q. How do you know it was a migraine and not a headache?

A. [Mother] The way he described the pain was exactly the same type as the migraines I get so I knew straight away what it was.

Q. How long have you and his father been separated?

A. [Mother] approximately two years

Q. Does he come home sick regularly after seeing his father?

A. [Mother] No.

Q. Does he get along well with his father?

A. [Mother] His dad doesn't understand him. He doesn't understand that he is special – he is sensitive and requires a different sort of approach. His father is blunt and doesn't realise how hurtful some of the things he says about T C can be.

Q. In what way is he sensitive?

A. [Mother] He takes things to heart and is easily upset by any criticism and takes everything that everyone has to say personally.

Q. [To TC] How do you get on at school?

A. It's all right. Some of the classes are good.

Q. Do you have many friends?

A. I have one.

Q. What do you do at lunchtime and recess with your friend?

A. We just talk or go somewhere quiet.

Q. Do you join in and play games with the other kids?

A. No, the other kids don't like me much.

[Mother] He gets picked on at school and we have an issue of bullying at the moment that has reached a point where I am thinking of changing schools.

Q. [To TC] What do these boys do to you?

A. They are not all boys, some are girls as well.

Q. Do they tease you or physically hurt you or both?

A. Most of the time they just tease me and call me names but sometimes they punch me as well.

TC begins to cry at this point.

[Mother] He thinks differently to the other kids. He thinks on a grand scale. For example last night he was talking about different strategies for solving poverty in the third world. It worries him that there are other children that don't have enough to eat or are dying of starvation. He saw a program on landmines which showed children his own age, some without any legs and it made a deep impression on him.

Q. Apart from the migraines do you have any other complaints?

A. Sometimes I feel like I'm going to be sick for no reason.

Q. Do you vomit?

A. No, never, but if I feel sick in the morning it will stay with me right up until I go to bed that day.

Q. Do you often have a headache with it?

A. No but sometimes I am very sleepy and tired.

[Mother] His energy levels are not good. He always is complaining of being tired no matter how much sleep he gets.

Q. Is he a nervous child?

A. [Mother] Yes very, particularly with noise.

Q. [To TC] What about music, do you like music?

A. No, it all sounds like clatter and noise and it gives me a headache.

Q. Do you play sport?

A. I don't like sports.

Q. Why not?

A. Because I'm not any good at them.

   The rubrics chosen for the case were:

   HEAD PAIN; LOCALISATION; sides; right.

   HEAD PAIN; PULSATING, throbbing.

   MIND; SENSITIVE, oversensitive; music, to.

   MIND; SENSITIVE, oversensitive; noise, to.

   MIND; AILMENTS from; reproaches.

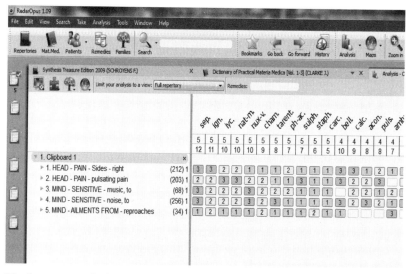

Under normal circumstances Carcinosin would be the number one choice repertorising so highly for a remedy found in less rubrics.

Facial features

Yellow

Widow's peak in the hairline

Down turned sloping eyes

Freckles

Red

Wide mouth

Full lips

Top of ears pinned back

This gives us a total of three yellows and three reds making T C orange. Our orange choices from this repertorisation include Ignatia, Nux Vom. and Nat Mur. Nat Mur. was chosen and 200C given.

Two weeks later no migraines. One month later no migraines and has made another friend at school. He is not being picked on as much. Two months later no migraines and now has a small group of friends and is not being picked on at school.

THE GENERALS OF ORANGE

AGGRAVATIONS

Anger

Emotions

Fatigue(burn out)

Wind

Extremes of temperature

Lying down

Attention

Disappointed love

Grief

Music

Worry

Noise

Milk

Coffee

Stimulants

Alcohol

AMELIORATIONS

Motion

Hard pressure

Gentle motion

Support

Milk

Open air

SENSATIONS

Bitter

Nausea

Cramping

Spasms

Intolerable

Plug

Numb

Oversensitive to pain

Throbbing

Echo

Needle like

Nail

Contraction

Twitching

Burning

Salty

FOOD

Desires acids/sour

Thirstless

Aggravation coffee

Desires and aggravation from bread and other starchy foods

Aversion to fats, rich foods and meat

Aggravation alcohol

Aversion to hot drinks

SEX

Retroverted uterus

Prolapses

Aversion to coition

Dysmenorrhoea

Tendency to abortion

Ovarian cyst

Dark menses

Frigidity

Premature ejaculation

Excessive milk

PATHOLOGY

Angina. Vision disturbances. Eye problems. **Squints. Neuralgia. Liver.** Low blood pressure. High blood pressure. **Fainting.** Anaemia. **Rheumatism.** Candida. **Thrush. Cold sores. Gallstones. Gout. Palpitations.** Arrhythmia. **Jaw problems. Sinus.** Irritable bowel syndrome. **Allergic reactions to insect bites.** Local inflammations. **Prolapses.** Uterine displacements. **Miscarriage. General lack of tone.** Cramps. **Colic. Paralysis**

of single parts. Nausea. **Acidic constitutions. Dysmenorrhea. Spasms. Teething Bronchitis. Insomnia**. Nervous exhaustion. Vertigo.

CHAPTER 18

Miasmatic Themes - Syco-Syphilis (Purple)

P ower is an aphrodisiac."

Like all the miasms, purple has a vast array of potential expressions. Again like every miasmatic group, we will be discussing the various themes that have arisen via clinical consultations. A miasmatic theme is discovered by observing repeating patterns in the stories presented by patients who respond well to purple remedies. After a number of patients have been treated, it becomes obvious that their stories show a remarkable similarity. Once a theme can be seen, other aspects of a case can also be examined to see what other themes might be common to the group. A theme is a story or event that occurs more often within one miasmatic group than would otherwise be expected. For example a strong sexual element exists within purple. However while sex is a primary driving force, it does not mean that it will be a problem area or of primary concern to every patient. However, for many, sex is a major issue and may direct the consultation, whether it is the pursuit of some specific sexual preference or a complete absence or denial of it. Either way sexual issues are an area of enormous importance and in far greater statistical numbers to purple than in patients from any other miasm.

Perhaps the strong sexual component of purple can be best understood by the need to be loved and desired given to it by red combined with the perversity and dysfunctional element supplied by blue. Hence sexual dysfunction is a strong theme in this group. This combination of a high sex drive from red with the obsessional or dysfunctional property of blue, accounts for rubrics such as the "pederasty" and "sodomy" of Platina, the masochism of Lachesis or the complete aversion to sex as noted in Staphisagria. The form sexual desire or sexual preference may take is as varied as there are people on the planet so one cannot put forward statements like "The sexual preference of purple is ..." When dealing with miasmatic themes we are dealing with patterns and tendencies not exact events, therefore the amount of times sex presents itself as an issue is the real indicator of its energetic significance. All miasms have a strong sexual element in them, but a strong and healthy sex drive is different from a decided preoccupation.

TERROR, TORMENT AND PANIC

A common and prominent problem area for purple is their tendency to panic attacks and anxiety disorders. Purple is not the only miasmatic group to have panic attacks but they are certainly more prone to them than most. Only brown has more nervous disorders than this miasm. Many display a type of behaviour consistent with being on red alert. Seeing danger everywhere many are on a constant vigil to protect themselves from those who would hurt or take advantage of them.

The type of panic attack purple is likely to suffer is where the patient needs to stop the car. They feel like they are having a heart attack because of the chest pain, their face becomes pale, their perspiration cold. Life and everything in it stops at this point and any thought of pushing through the pain barrier is completely out of the question. The patient is completely frozen in time and space and all that is important is surviving the next second. Everything is bleak, hopeless and frightening. It is pointless continuing any further as everything is futile. They are completely irrational.

In some respects their whole life can be a subclinical version of such a panic attack – the same sentiments, at a continuous but much lower pitch. The strain, the terror, the suspicion and the vulnerability all combined with a demanding, aggressive but hysterical attitude completes the picture of purple.

MIND; DELUSIONS, imaginations; deserted, forsaken.

MIND; DELUSIONS, imaginations; doomed, being.

MIND; MANIA, madness; rage, with.

SUSPICION, HATRED AND VICTIMISATION

With nervous systems consistently on guard and ready for attack, purple will launch at anyone who threatens them. Purple eyes can see enemies everywhere, no one can be thoroughly trusted. As a defence a brazen and swaggering attitude may be adopted, a "too cool for school" posture designed to make people too nervous to try anything. Unfortunately it often serves to bring loathing from some quarters together with a desire to "cut them down to size". The very thing they believe everyone is trying to do, becomes self fulfilling due to their defensive actions. Remedies such as Lachesis, Platina and Veratrum all have an air of arrogance and one-upmanship about them. They also carry a strong level of attack and violence. However this can also go the opposite way, and as a defence some may become sweet and pliable as seen in Staphisagria, or extravagant and spoiling with their affection. None the less the air of violence and "rip off" is around them. One can only see and recognise in others what is present within us. Purple evoke the Napoleonic standpoint that the best form of defence is attack, and as a consequence may be seen by others as the perpetrator rather than someone who is defending themselves. They may feel perfectly justified "getting in first", protecting themselves and their possessions. Even though it is they that started the attack, some can be completely surprised if not downright shocked that someone could dare accuse *them* of being the bad one. In their eyes, you would have done exactly the same thing had you had the foresight and wisdom to see what was around the corner, their accuser is just jealous they did not get in first, "They have no right to scold me simply because I got what I wanted and they did not".

Purple rarely, if ever see themselves as the "bad guy" no matter how hurtful their actions may be. Life is a do or die competition for survival, and they just happen to be better at it than the next person. No amount of explanation is sufficient to make them understand they were unjustified in doing what they did to their partner, friend or sibling. Why should they be penalised for doing what was going to be done to them only they didn't give the other person the chance? Any sanction against them is unjustified and unfair and only serves to re-enforce their belief that everyone is against them and trying to get at them. People are ready to band together like a lynch mob for the sole purpose of bringing them down for nothing more than the satisfaction they gain from being nasty to them.

Anyone who tries to harm, suppress or stand in their way does so because they hate them and has a vendetta against them. People are *always* taking someone else's side because everyone hates them, so purple vows to hate them back. They often feel victimised, whether from paranoia or reality.

Purple can be intellectually or emotionally immature. As well as arrogant many are also dependent, a reason they can habitually attempt to capitalise at another's expense in seemingly cruel and underhanded ways, never acknowledging personal responsibility but rather defending their actions vehemently. Any attempt to modify, punish or counsel will be deemed as a meddlesome attempt to regulate based on the fact that the person enforcing the discipline is doing so because they hate them.

Delusion and reality are two sides of the same energetic coin and as a consequence anyone belonging to this miasm may only be a knife's edge away from the real hatred and violence that accompanies it. The potential of this miasm shows its presence in stories of continuous abuse and victimisation.

The abuse most suffered in purple will be sexual, as there is a great deal of sexual energy around them. There can be more than one perpetrator and it can occur in unrelated time frames and ways. Without a knowledge of miasmatic energy one is at a complete loss to understand how one person can suffer so much abuse throughout their lifetime.

If I see you as my enemy then I will treat you as such. You in turn will respond to the way I treat you by treating me as an enemy and will behave in the same hostile way I treated you. Which one is real, the belief that you are an enemy or the fact that now you are one? The difference between belief and actuality is non-existent for whilst my delusion to treat you as an enemy was not justified, your response to my attitude confirms that it was. Once you become my enemy, my original delusion is reality and as a consequence not a delusion at all.

In homoeopathy it is the energy that is real; this is the force we deal with. Like an aura, it precedes and determines the form and function of the matter that will eventually grow into it. The miasmatic energy that an individual brings with them into the world will determine the events and circumstances that will take place within the course of their lives. Not at any moment can the observer be separated from the observed. The victim and the perpetrator are as energetically linked as any other web of life. This neither excuses nor blames, but it does help to understand what lies behind. It may at first seem trite to explain events as purple or blue or green, as if in some way that is a reason something has occurred, but, once understood, it is in fact the most comprehensive of explanations.

MIND; DELUSIONS, imaginations; injury; injured, is being.

MIND; DELUSIONS, imaginations; pursued, he is.

MIND; CRUELTY, brutality, inhumanity.

MIND; MISANTHROPY.

MIND; VIOLENCE, vehemence; deeds of, rage leading to.

HAUGHTINESS, CONTEMPT AND ARROGANCE

Sometimes believed sometimes bravado, purple may have an

arrogance that can extend into contempt. Most homoeopaths are experienced in the conceit of Lachesis or Platina, but it is important to understand that this attitude belongs to purple as a general theme. When repertorising a purple case, haughtiness and arrogance are much less enticing rubrics to choose due to its "genus epidemicus" status. To see a patient put on such a strong persona is to recognise that, other symptoms agreeing, this is simply purple at work. This point is driven home when, as a practitioner, you bear witness to the same story being told over and over again by different patients. What emotional or mental residue is left behind after an event accounts for why an array of medicines from each miasmatic family is needed. Each medicine has a slight variance that separates it from all the others from within its family.

One homoeopathic medicine can never do the work of another. As an example, a person who is confident, perhaps even arrogant, around their family and friends is only in such a position of power while everyone agrees to treat them as such. But should someone decide to take them to task, to expose or belittle them, their standing may be damaged beyond repair. If this patient had presented to our clinic before their loss of face perhaps Lachesis or Platina would have been the remedy of choice, but if they were to turn up after, then remedies like Staphisagria may come to the fore.

MIND; RUDENESS.

MIND; INSOLENCE, impertinence.

MIND; CONTEMPTUOUS.

MIND; DELUSIONS, imaginations; great person, is.

SEX, PERVERSITY AND COMMUNICATION

Highly sexed and highly communicative are two accurate descriptors for purple. It is no coincidence that remedies such as Lachesis, Hyoscyamus and Stramonium feature as some of the main remedies for loquaciousness, and also have a strong sexual component. Sex, another form of expressive communication, can also be, like its verbal counterpart, rapid, hectic and loquacious. The sexual impulse of purple can be driving and unquenchable. Occasionally this drive may be fuelled by an inability to gain satisfactory release.

Sexual dysfunction in purple ranges from extreme promiscuity to total abstinence, from never being satisfied to unenjoyable, it may also include self-harm, masochism, incest and pederasty. Purple is the miasm most prone to sexual abuse as they have a strong sexual energy, but this is due to inheritance, which means someone else in their household may also have a strong but perverse sexual drive. This can be disastrous.

Self-mutilation, whether for sexual gratification or not, can be a strong but not exclusive indicator for this miasm. Sexual dysfunction combines with another typically purple trait, better by discharges or flow, to mould a sexual appetite for pain. To draw blood and gain release or to use the same as a sexual stimulant is not uncommon.

Sexual energy is not always applied negatively, indeed the miasm may be displayed in an entirely different way, leaving their sexual side unencumbered. There are also some who have a strong sexual presence but none of the dysfunction. Rather than being targeted they may have such a presence that others are falling at their feet just to be close to them. Rather than tragic, they become erotic and glamorous.

MIND; LEWDNESS, obscene.

MIND; DELIRIUM; erotic.

MIND; AMATIVENESS.

RELIGION, SPIRITUALITY AND THE SUPERNATURAL

Probably the most common theme running through purple is religion and/or spirituality. Purple is the chosen colour for many religious denominations and is the colour of preference for many new-age spiritual philosophies. Whether in the priesthood or in magic, purple symbolises a degree of spiritual attainment and signifies an elevated level of evolvement. For novice and serious advocate, the range of mystic traditions they may be drawn into is vast. It may be a traditional belief system like Catholicism or it may be a personalised conglomeration of various beliefs.

Magic can play a part in their life as may conspiracy theories. Indeed conspiracies can be viewed as a type of similimum for purple. For example, conspiracies fuel suspicion. Conspiracy theories imply that you are now part of a small sanctum of people that know something others do not, satisfying their haughtiness. Lastly, conspiracy theories suit purple as they are based on the belief that "everyone is trying to get you".

This suspicion sometimes combines with their sexual energy to create rubrics like, "Delusions, that their wife is being unfaithful", and "Jealousy during drunkenness". Suspicion and infidelity surrounds them, they see it everywhere because it is in them.

Clairvoyance features as does clairaudience and divination. Sometimes however these abilities can be anything but helpful and may leave their host feeling tormented and schizophrenic. When pushed to extremes, some talk of being damned or knowing that hell and all it has to offer awaits, all salvation is lost. Under "anxiety about salvation" three of the five **bold** remedies are purple; Lachesis, Staphisagria and Veratrum Album.

MIND; DELUSIONS, imaginations; devils.

MIND; DELUSIONS, imaginations; religious.

MIND; INSANITY, madness; religious.

GREED

In the Buddhist tradition the flaw of greed would sit most comfortably with purple. In this sense greed differs from the desire of orange in that it attempts to capitalise at the expense of another. There is no room for second place with greed. To come second is to be first loser. Their world is one where the winner takes it all and they can get malicious if they think they will miss out. Purple can and will share with others, indeed quite lavishly, but this is only after *their* needs and wishes have been gratified. Sometimes done in the true spirit of giving and sometimes done to try and win back favour after having treated others badly, purple can and do bestow presents and attention to those they choose and nobody does it more elaborately. Most are only venomous when they believe they are being attacked or when they think they will miss out. It is hardly surprising then that material gain is a prime motivation for this miasm. Goods and chattels are benchmarks of self-worth. They can be driven to succeed, finding themselves in positions of great wealth and power. The halls of power, or even more likely, the power and money that finance the halls of power, probably contain a disproportionate number of purple members. They are strong, wilful and focused. In business they turn their suspicion into cunning, their arrogance into confidence and their contemptuous attitude into a type of currency that buys the admiration of those around them. They have an ability to be one step ahead, to see things coming before rather than after an event. Many are prepared to do what it takes to get the job done. They can be audacious and bold, prepared to take risks. Their decision-making, like their spending, is extravagant. Above all other miasmatic groups they can walk that fine line between supreme hero and supreme villain. To them dreams are futile unless they materialise into fact. In this mode, purple are charismatic, they stand out, they are distinct and fascinating and they are extremely intelligent. Powerful, confident, charismatic and sexual, these are all purple qualities, a gifted combination when used wisely.

People such as this are idolised, fawned over, looked upon as winners – they are larger than life. They deserve all the perks that big money can bestow because they have earned them. At this stage the story comes full circle as arrogance reigns and underlings grovel and creep to their higher purple masters.

So far purple has been examined in regards to how it will present itself most commonly in the clinic, but like all patients some will present with little if any real structural pathology. This means their miasm is being constructively utilised, for pathology is always in direct proportion to happiness. The happier a person is, the less pathology they have. The more mentally or emotionally tortured they are, the more structurally malfunctioning their body.

When is someone happy? There are two answers:

1. When their miasmatic demands are being gratified. (pleasure)

2. When miasmatic demands have been transcended. (happiness)

The problem with answer one is that it is temporary, naïve, bereft and ultimately futile.

The problem with answer two is that it's hard to achieve*.

Purple patients with little if any pathology are like people from any other miasmatic group whose life is going according to their wishes. They are happy, contented and self-satisfied. The problem for purple is that of all the miasmatic groups, it is they who are dominated by greed and this places contentedness further from their reach than any other miasms.

> * Footnote 2008 Rather than transcendence or gratification, contentment and happiness comes from the understanding of our base desires in balance with our higher ideals, as further discussed in **Soul & Survival (2008)**

CHILDISHNESS

Described by Max Luscher discussing the psychology of colours he writes:

The preference for violet among pre-adolescents highlights the fact that, to them, the world is still a magical place in which they only have to rub Aladdin's lamp for its slave to bring them what they want ...

The childishness of purple lies in their inability to progress beyond the adolescent. Their tendency to remain in this selfish and demanding stage is too strong. Like most adolescents many will insist on all the benefits and none of the responsibilities – this makes them reliant on someone else to do all their dirty work. Like an adolescent they begrudge their dependence and often take out their more than ample frustrations on those whom they are most dependent upon. As a consequence temper tantrums can result no matter what the age. In more mature years it will manifest itself more as manipulation than outright bullying, but it is a tantrum, none the less, no matter how sophisticated its presentation.

Relationships will be another area where purple childishness can show itself. Often a relationship is seen as something you draw from as opposed to something you jointly give to. "What can I get out of this relationship?" may hold precedence over, "How I feel about you?"

Childishness can exhibit itself via inappropriate behaviour. Laughing at serious times, or too loudly. Symptoms such as these are a direct consequence of their emotional immaturity. An inability to grasp more refined and subtle emotional concepts may lead others to believe they are insensitive and uncaring; neither may be true, most times they are actually missing what is going on. They may understand when they have the problem explained to them, but it must be in a way they can understand. They may be highly intelligent, but some have the emotional understanding of a twelve-year-old.

Purple may be completely unprepared to make the necessary commitment needed to make a relationship work. Their relationship is often based on taking, not giving, or the opposite of all giving and no taking, which is just as immature. Some may be left by their partner on the basis they are simply too demanding, while others are abused and walked over. Many times I have seen purple partner with brown, as only brown is prepared to give to the level required by purple. They may need and rely on their brown partner but may not love or respect them, and as a consequence may treat their brown partner abominably.

VIOLENCE AND SELF-DESTRUCTIVE BEHAVIOUR

Even though the "violent" aspect of purple stems from its blue parentage, the aggressive outward targeting of it has been given by red. As a result purple can exhibit both outward as well as self-abusing violent behaviour. Violence projected outwardly needs little explanation in regards to tell-tale signs, but self-directed violence can often take some tricky and deceiving turns. The most common forms of self abuse purple are likely to inflict include:

1. Alcohol and drug addiction

Many seem particularly prone to drug addiction.

MIND; MORPHINISM, drug addiction.

2. Self-mutilation

Seen mainly under times of stress this form of abuse is not suicidal nor is it an attempt to try and brand themselves. It is a release from pressure achieved through pain or blood flow. Patients will describe how they burn themselves with cigarettes, sew their fingers together, or cut themselves with knives or bottles when they become angry or frustrated. The relief gained from this behaviour is only temporary but still the temptation seems too great for some to conquer.

3. Anorexia and bulimia

A common form of self-abuse for this miasm.

4. Promiscuousness

Whether or not this is to be regarded as destructive behaviour depends on the motivating drive behind it, and how they feel about the event afterwards. Purple may also use sex as a weapon in a power play with their partner.

SWEETNESS

In contrast, some will try and quell the aggression or chaos going on around them by being as sweet as possible. They are gentle and may act as a moderator to the aggressive energies that exist around them. They are nice people who those that will mistreat them or threaten them, they are always placating the fury, turning a blind eye or more commonly bearing the brunt. This type seem infinite in their acceptance of the misbehaviour of their partner, and rather than applauded they are sacrificed. Staphisagria get their deserved reputation for exploding with anger after the remedy because of this trait. In some ways this can be similar to brown but underneath there is an anger or a revenge that brown is less likely to have.

CASE 1 – Ms M aged thirty

Presenting with diagnosed irritable bowel syndrome. Features of case include:

Burning and twisting sensations in the transverse colon.

Stress.

History of hay fever and occasional slight asthma.

History of Bells palsy.

History of acne.

IBS symptoms include:

Aggravation from dairy products like milk which creates a burning sensation as soon as it hits the stomach.

Aggravation from beer and wine.

Aggravation from stress.

Aggravation from anger.

Ms M describes herself as easygoing, a good talker and communicator which is her strongest asset. She is the daughter of a very successful father whom she described as pushy and overbearing.

"No one could have a say while he was around, he was continuously trying to get both myself and my brother into the family business. If I even suggested that my talents may lie elsewhere he would respond with ridicule jumping in quickly to point out that I had no talents. I once replied to him that if I am so talentless why do you want me as an employee, to which he responded with such a verbal tirade that all future discussions became pointless. He was constantly driving me, all through school and college he would pressure me. He can be very dominating and very critical. He throws fits if he does not get what he wants".

Q. How did this make you feel about yourself and your place in the family?

A. I was very angry most of the time, I used to storm to my room to escape literally trembling with anger, how dare he treat me that way!! He showed no respect for me, I would be furious!

Q. You haven't mentioned your mother.

A. No, she was all right, in the end she became a hermit – almost, I still see her, she's OK.

Q. Why is your IBS so bad at the moment? Is there anything stressful going on in your life?"

A. Work is stressful. At the moment the company I work for is cutting back on staff. They have been doing so for the past six weeks. Nobody knows what their future is. Every Friday they call one or two people into the office and tell them not to bother to turn up Monday. It's cruel the way they are going about it.

Q. What emotions have arisen most in you during the last six weeks?

A. Anger, sometimes to the point where I just think I am going to explode, how dare they treat us with so little respect, to humiliate us all in such a fashion, if there was something I could do about it I would, but there just isn't anything. I am completely powerless, I just have to sit and wait like everyone else.

The rubrics chosen for her case included

MIND; AILMENTS from indignation.

GENERALITIES; FOOD and drinks; beer; agg.

MIND; AILMENTS from; anger, vexation.

GENERALITIES; FOOD and drinks; wine; agg.

GENERALITIES; FOOD and drinks; milk; agg.

ABDOMEN; PAIN; twisting.

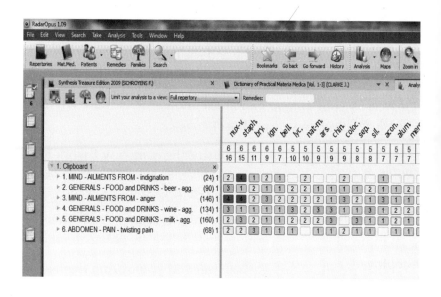

Facial features

Yellow

Bump on the bone of the nose (profile)

Red

Protruding eyes (exopthalmic)

Straight hairline

Full lips

Full smile

Blue

Asymmetry - nose and chin

Dimples

Recessed lids

The summary of her facial features were; 4 red, 3 blue and 1 yellow. There is obviously not enough yellow in her facial structure to make her brown but the near even amount of red to blue features leaves little doubt that she is purple.

In this repertorisation there are only two purple remedies; Staphisagria and Belladonna. Obviously Staphisagria is the remedy of choice and was given in the 10M potency.

I did not see Ms M for another seven months when her IBS trouble was just beginning to return. According to Ms M the medicine had worked almost immediately. Staphisagria 10M was repeated, again with instant results.

As a footnote Ms M was not sacked from her job but was redeployed into another area; she is content with this outcome and enjoys her new role.

CASE 2 – Mr K aged forty

Diagnosed with fibromyalgia. Complaints include muscle aches and pains, lethargy and heartburn. He has been putting on a great deal of weight over recent months even though his diet is much the same as it ever was.

He also has insomnia, and suffers from night terrors that leave him with a sense of nothingness.

He has a great deal of lower back pain < right to left, < lying down.

Burning pain in his rib cage; pain goes from right to left.

Wakes during the night – possibly around 2.00 a.m.?

Very bad heartburn < lying down.

Throbbing pain in sternum < lying down.

Occasional nausea especially with the heartburn.

Q. What features or traits do you have that individualise you from others?

A. I often know what is going to happen before an event takes place.

Q. You're clairvoyant?

A. I'm not sure about that, it's not like I can do it at will or anything, but every now and then I will get these strong déjà vu feelings, to the point where I can tell who is going to say what next.

Q. Does this happen with events also? And is it always related to you or can it be more general?

A. No it can definitely be more general, I have dreamt some world events sometimes up to months before they occur.

Q. You said earlier that you had night terrors where there was nothing but emptiness, can you tell me a little more about this feeling?

A. I don't know what else to say, they are terrifying, you are detached and there is nothing, like astral travelling except you don't see anything.

Q. You astral travel?

A. Not very often. I first realised I could do it after I had what I would call a near psychotic breakdown after smoking hashish with some friends. Since then I have separated from my body on a number of occasions, at first I thought I was made schizophrenic from the drugs, it was very scary and I took a vow never to take drugs again – which I have stuck to. I also do not drink alcohol very much as I can get mean, alcohol is very bad for my personality.

Q. You said earlier that clairvoyance only happened few and far between, what about astral travel?

A. I can do that very easily – it is now at the point where I can separate from my body almost anytime I want to, it is no longer scary, now it is fun.

Q. What aspects of your character do you think could use a little improvement?

A. I can be terribly outspoken and critical. Impatience is my absolute worst feature, if something isn't done in the time frame I want – look out. I have a very bad temper and can be vindictive; if someone gets me, I will get them back ten times harder.

The rubrics chosen for his case were

STOMACH; HEARTBURN.

GENERALITIES; SIDE; right; left, then.

MIND; CLAIRVOYANCE.

MIND; DELUSIONS, imaginations; soul; body is too small for, or that it is separated from.

MIND; IMPATIENCE.

GENERALITIES; LYING; agg.

GENERALITIES; FOOD and drinks; alcohol, alcoholic drinks; agg.

GENERALITIES; SIDE; right.

GENERALITIES; PAIN; burning; internally.

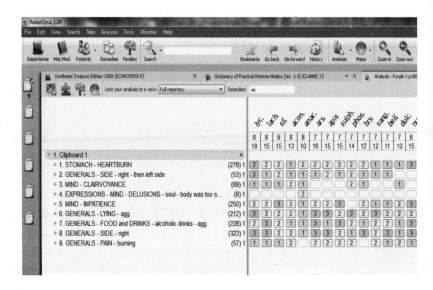

An equal distribution of both red and blue exists in this patient. There was no recognisable yellow in his facial structure.

Facial features

Red

Lines - brackets

Wide nose

Single line

Blue

Wide-set eyes

Set-back hairline

Inward angle of the teeth

The major decision in this repertorisation was between Belladonna and Anacardium. Anacardium 1M was chosen because of its potential harshness and because it is the only purple remedy listed for the delusion that his soul is separated from his body.

Three weeks later his report was that his back and muscle aches were better and all his heartburn was gone. He had not chosen to astral travel during this time period as he had made a conscious decision that he should try harder to be happier down here on earth.

Six months later some heartburn began to return and he recently had a bad nightmare. Anacardium 1M was repeated.

THE GENERALS OF PURPLE

SENSATIONS

Trembling

Plug

Lump

Twitching

Constriction

Squeezing

Cold

Numbness

FOOD

Aggravation or amelioration – fruits

Aggravation – coffee

Alcohol and sweets

AGGRAVATIONS AND AMELIORATIONS

Aversion water/fluids

Aggravation before menstruation

Sleep/after sleep

Disappointed love

Sexual desire

PATHOLOGY

Insomnia. **Panic attacks. Cancer** and malignancies. **Gangrene.**
Hyperthyroid. **Epilepsy.** Hyper activity. Menopause problems.
Nail biting. Nervous breakdown. Pre-menstrual syndrome. Root
canal. Stuttering. **Teeth**. Throat. Tinnitus. Urinary infections.
Endocrine dysfunction. Nightmares. **Night terrors.**

CHAPTER 19

Miasmatic Themes - Tubercular (Green)

From looking at several copies of the portraits of Samuel Hahnemann it seems likely he belonged to this miasmatic group. The curved domed forehead of blue combined with the down-turned eyes of yellow. However his eyes are also quite deep set (blue), he had a small thin mouth (yellow) a deeply indented bridge of the nose (blue) as well as having the yellow bump in the nose often giving it a hooked curvature. All this is purely speculative of course and portraits vary considerably, nonetheless those facial structures are the most commonly reproduced features in the majority of his portraits.

Consider also the following quote with Hahnemann in mind.

Green as tension therefore acts as a dam behind which the excitation of external stimuli builds up without being released, increasing the sense of pride, of self-controlled superiority over others, of power, of being in control of events, or at least of being able to manage and direct them. This damming-up and suppression of external stimuli lead to many forms and degrees of "control", not only in the sense of directed drives, but also as detailed accuracy in checking and verifying facts, as precise and accurate memory, as clarity of presentation, critical analysis and logical consistency –

all the way up to abstract formalism. This "green" behaviour can also find expression in a quest for better conditions, such as improved health, or a longer more useful life both for him and for others. In this case we have the reformer, bent on ameliorating conditions.

Green has an arrogance that can only be matched by purple. Hahnemann had a self-assuredness that consistently placed him in positions of trouble. If Hahnemann was in fact green, this is hardly surprising, as no miasmatic group is more combative and downright contrary than this. To outsiders it can sometimes seem as if they deliberately go out of their way to cause trouble. Whenever Mother Nature decides that things are becoming complacent and a stir of the pot is needed, for better or worse it will often be a green she sends down.

Whether or not Hahnemann was truly green will never be known but it is safe to say that his life story was dominated by a green energy to the point that his biography is a good, if not somewhat exaggerated example of what this energy is capable of.

Hahnemann was critical and scathing of anyone for whom he had professional contempt. His passionate outbursts and fiery temperament in defence of homoeopathy were legendary. He was persecuted and ridiculed, continuously moving. Never resting, Hahnemann kept experimenting, discovering deeper insights into homoeopathy always mesmerised by what he found; the thrill never left him. Outside of his profession and certainly towards his patients, his tolerance and acceptance were boundless. But to those within the profession, if they showed ignorance or laziness of any kind or ridiculed his system, he was merciless in his counterattack. Hahnemann was clear, critical and detailed, he was indeed a reformer who knew he was right, if the rest of the world did not agree with him, then the rest of the world was wrong. In his personal life he seems to have been well liked, not just respected for his achievements. Last, but not least, in a typically green fashion, Hahnemann always had people around him who cared for him and assisted him in every way possible, whether it was his daughters, his first wife whom he openly admits did virtually everything for him, or Melanie who took him to Paris and made sure he received the respect and prestige that was owed. This green need to have someone around to take on the practical responsibilities of life is ever present. Just as an artist needs a patron to finance them and give them the independence required to do their work, so too do many greens need a helping hand in matters practical. Very few greens can make it on their own; being alone is what they are worst at. Green is always ready to hand over the reins of a task they find monotonous, not because they're lazy, although that may be part of it, but because they have an all or nothing aspect to their character. This means that many can be accomplished, even experts in a given area, but completely incompetent outside of it. They may be the tradesman who can turn their hand to anything but has never had a deep conversation in their life, or a musician who would get regular work if they would just remember to turn up once in a while.

These extremes or opposites stem from the fact that both yellow and blue are literally poles apart; even red and blue are closer and have more in common. These two miasms, psora and syphilis, are the yin and the yang of the homoeopathic world. Introspective and deep (blue) but sunny and light (yellow), needing to withdraw from everyone (blue) but at the same time much worse for it (yellow). Constantly on the move either mentally or physically, green goes through their whole life swinging from hot to cold and back again. Easily bored, they will go from one subject or project to the other. They are a walking inconsistency because of these two opposing miasms; therefore the energy around them will also be in constant disagreement.

FEAR, STRESS AND ESCAPE

There is a strong potential for stress in this miasm. Whenever blue is joined to any colour it magnifies its co-tenant's qualities to even greater levels than the miasm it originated from. For example, red may have suspicion but purple or brown may have paranoia. Yellow has fear and anxiety and so in consequence, green may be subject to levels of stress that would constitute a nervous breakdown. The blue part of green prevents them dropping the anxiety and moving on to other things, even long after the actual stress has passed. Their initial reaction to stress is often either a frenetic tirade of abuse, accusations and threats or an immediate reliance on someone around them to take over and relieve them of the burden. More often than not, this stress will come from outside their area of expertise making them feel inept at dealing with it. Some, once reassured that everything will be all right, will finally begin to calm down and relax, others are not so easily swayed, can carry the stress for an eternity, needing positive reassurance over and over again. In stress, areas like in many other areas of their life, green may need continuous propping–up.

Phosphorus has a reputation for being able to tell the mood of a room the moment they walk into it, but many belonging to this miasm that are not Phosphorus have this same sensitivity. Green needs constant stimulation, praise and reassurance from those around them if they are to successfully navigate their way through life; many are totally dependent on the skills and friendship of others.

Stress is not good for anybody's health, but here it causes

more suffering than most, indeed Phosphorus itself is the only remedy in the rubric, "MIND; CARES, worries; full of; constitution, undermined by".

Because it already contains two extremes, to add another, in any form, may quickly tip them over the edge. Some go into an instant frenzy, while others need dead quiet and calm to think before they act, either way the pressure must stop before any positive response can occur.

If stress becomes prolonged or insurmountable their first instinctive reaction is to head for the hills and put as much distance as possible between them and the problem. In regards to the two most basic stress responses, fight or flight, green instinctively chooses flight. Some as a compensation may train themselves in the area of fight, to overcome their flight like the temper and desire to fight exhibited by Tuberculinum but more often than not they will talk of how, all they want to do is pack it all in and move away to somewhere exotic so they don't have to worry about such stupid little details ever again. No such place on God's earth exists but it is still what they desire.

Panic and terror and the need for constant reassurance come from the giving ground and collapse of blue. Eventually though, their yellow survival side will kick in, and enough will be enough, a solution must be sought.

MIND; Fits of violent temper; wants to fight.

MIND; CARES, worries; full of; constitution, undermined by.

DISSATISFACTION AND PERFECTION

The most well-known of all the tubercular traits, dissatisfaction, is constant because of the pull between the two distinct but opposing miasms. What will satisfy at one point of time will not suffice at another, how could it when the two miasmatic demands are conflicting? This leaves many in a position of always feeling empty or unfulfilled; to them, no matter how good an event, it could have been better. Rarely do they ever have that 'simply perfect' feeling. As a consequence, many are on the lookout for an excuse, a cause, something or someone that is stopping things from being perfect. In their mind if this could be eradicated everything would be ideal. This means green is continually finding a cause or enemy on whom to redirect their energy. In an Orwellian fashion, war, by finding an external enemy, creates peace by having an excuse to legitimise their dissatisfaction; hence someone, or something, is always in the gun. Almost impossible to please when they reach this level green can be ferocious and infuriating, critical of everything and everyone.

Another way dissatisfaction may show itself is in the vacillation of its own desires. Manifested in their sexual life where their desire for something exotic and different may only be surpassed by their fear of getting it. This springs from their famous "grass is greener" attitude to life. Firstly they want something, then they don't, then they do again and then when they get it it's the wrong sort or colour or type. Yearning for something that they can't handle or don't really want makes those around them fed up, cross and impatient. Green in turn gets hurt and defensive. Because of their focus on what is *not* right, the slightest thing that goes wrong in their plan is focused upon and magnified out of all proportion.

They are demanding in regards to their environment; they crave aesthetic beauty because it is perfect. Green is demanding of their partners, and demanding of themselves. With such an eye for beauty and perfection, they may put themselves through torture to get their project "just right". They will labour for hours to get a picture, engine or sentence exactly the way they want it. They are not perfectionists per se, as rarely does this sort of effort and detail extend beyond what they are passionate about. Being so exacting with themselves is why Hahnemann thought he had the right to condemn others who would dare focus on him when their own practices were so transparent and shoddy. A green in defence of their work is a green in full flight, and a green in full flight, as Hahnemann's reputation showed, is something to behold.

MIND; DESIRES; numerous and various things.

MIND; DESIRES; indefinite.

MIND; COMPLAINING.

POOR LEARNING SKILLS AND FEELING STUPID

Green more than any other miasmatic group has a disproportionate number of people who are right-brained. Perhaps this accounts for its artistic reputation? This means some are likely to develop at a much later stage. Many green children live in a dream world, escaping to some mental oasis when times get tough. Schooling is a predominantly left-brained affair; hence some green children find themselves left behind and it's at this stage that many become spiteful and rebellious. Knowing in their own minds they are not dull but being unable to academically prove it, they feel stupid.

Becoming deliberately contrary some develop bitterness, while others turn their attentions elsewhere, rejecting the system altogether. Contrariness and rebellion are part of their genetic miasmatic makeup, they are born to rebel; sometimes it just takes a while to find something to rebel against.

Just as Calc Carb. are late bloomers, not coming into their own until later on in life, the same can be applied for any remedy in the green miasmatic family. Continuing with Calc Carb. as an example, we see a person who is bright but not doing well at school, slower than their fellow students they are labelled as either lazy or dull, but green works on green time, push them and they will rebel. Many of this type would benefit from an alternative style of teaching; they will never fit into the conventional system. On the other side of the coin others are absolute academics, amassing a staggering array of knowledge and qualifications. They respond well to a system that provides everything, all they have to do is concentrate on the task at hand– this suits them perfectly. Indeed it may be so perfect they become a perpetual student. Whether mechanical, academic or abstract, the green mind is geared for creation, it is constantly developing new ideas, philosophies, inventions or machines.

The modern world is intolerant, ready to cut off at the knees anyone who does not conform quickly, so the more creative or abstract green may find, too late, that their future has been sealed, now locked into being a smart person in a dull job. A green case will often be filled with such things; responses of bitterness, lack of recognition, dignity and anger will feature prominently. Pride in their work or qualifications will also feature prominently. This scholastic type will take great pride in their academic achievements and give an air that makes others feel uneasy to be around. In this respect they may resemble purple in their arrogance and haughtiness, but usually it is just a hint of hubris, a subtle reminder of intellectual superiority rather than a coarse and "vulgar" display.

MIND; DISOBEDIENCE.

MIND; CONTRARY.

MIND; CONTRADICT, disposition to.

MIND; LEARNING; poorly.

IMPORTANCE AND RECOGNITION

It is vital to some to prove their worth, to become successful in their work. Unlike purple or yellow who will be driven by financial gains, green is often motivated by professional finesse and skill. Money is as important to them as it is to anyone else, survival and comfort depend on it, but rarely is it their prime motivator.

Some strive to place themselves into positions of importance within their field. Others will go into their own business, a synonym for their own world on their own terms. Here they can be left alone to do what they want in the time frame they want. Green is not a hermit by nature, Phosphorus is an example of that. Just as Phosphorus can be a social butterfly, so too can all greens. When upset they may scream they are going to leave every one behind and go off and find a cave somewhere, but the chances of them actually doing it are slim, for just as Calc withdraws into their hard shell, stubbornly clinging to the rock, so too will all this miasm at different times, but oysters live in colonies, and in the same way most greens, despite their protestations to the contrary, need company.

If a green does not develop their skill due to a lack of opportunity or sheer laziness, a few will try to win respect by claiming credit for things they didn't actually do; it is not beyond green to simply lie. To them it is important to be important and if they cannot do it by real achievements they may do it via false ones. They can deceive people by re-creating their past and exaggerating their skills or involvement, giving others the impression they have lived a life deserving of admiration when little if any of their story may be true. The only real truth is their ability for unbounded creativity and imagination, lies are just another expression of it.

Being desired is another way they can be recognised; some are flighty and flirtatious, going to whomever will give them the most attention. But obstinacy and willfulness are also part of the green make-up demonstrating their opposite ability to hold fast to commitments.

While not uncommon to be in charge of their project, it is rarer to find green in high management roles as this takes a level of multi-skilling that most do not have. It is also not suitable to their character. Unable to be told what to do, most have no burning desire to make a career out of telling others what to do. Green is after recognition not responsibility.

MIND; SELFISHNESS, egoism.

MIND; SYMPATHY, compassion; desire for. Consolation; amel.

RESPECT AND FREEDOM

These are two of their most important demands. Respect may come in the form of recognition, manners or etiquette. Some place enormous emphasis on manners and etiquette as they appreciate style and refinement. Enjoying the finer things of life and appreciating quality and beauty, some place great emphasis on style and are willing to pay an exorbitant price tag for anything that is defined as art, genius or novelty. Because they demand quality in themselves, they can see it in products or works of others. Some will not wear any article of clothing unless it is of high quality or exotic origins, regardless of whether they can afford it. This same theme will repeat itself in food, cars, holidays or partners.

Green may demand the freedom to do as they please. Intolerant of any suggestion of compromise, they fly into a tirade of abuse if disturbed, earning them a reputation for crankiness and exploding quickly. This does not mean they cannot be asked to help, quite the contrary, many have a nature that likes to contribute and are more than willing to pitch in, they just cannot be told when and how to do it.

MIND; TRAVEL; desire to.

MIND; ESCAPE, attempts to.

THE MEANING OF LIFE

Every miasm has its own unique outlook on spirituality even though not everyone within each miasm will be spiritual. Atheists belong to each miasmatic family, the difference will be why. A belief in God is not exclusive to any particular miasm, but interpretation of what God is will be. Green like many others can be drawn to the supernatural. There is an exoticism in the unknowable, an exuberance and exhilaration that only comes from a topic as extensive and awe-inspiring as the search for meaning. Because there is no tangible and concrete answer, all things are possible. Green is not trying to discover who they are like brown; most are trying to find out how it all works, the thinking behind it all. Green loves to be inspired and nothing can inspire them more than how the universe works. Green can have a fascination for anything that gives them a thrill, the supernatural both draws and scares them. To many nothing is more important than the mystery. If there is an actual answer I suspect many greens would be disappointed if they found it.

NOTHING FOR TOO LONG

Many have a personality that throws them into a task, but for the sake of their sanity, they will need to drop it from time to time and do something that is, in true green style, completely the opposite. They suffer burn-out easily and so diversion is an important part of their make-up. Like yellow or orange, green is easily bored as well as easily excitable. However because of the blue, green will be more explorative than yellow and less competent and structured than orange. Due to the yellow green is highly social and may have a diverse number of friends and social groups. Rather than having a close unchanging club of friends, they are more likely to have various groups representing their diverse range of interests; they will see each momentarily rather than one consistently.

MIND; IMPRESSIONABLE, susceptible.

MIND; ENNUI, boredom.

PRIDE AND ARTISTRY

Keeping with Buddhist descriptions, the vice that best sums up green is pride. This is why respect and recognition are such driving themes. It accounts for why they can be the most verbally vicious and condescending, and it accounts for why they critique everything and everyone. The green method of attack is to humiliate and ridicule, to make someone feel small and insignificant. When green decides to attack they will do so with scathing precision, telling you more about yourself than you knew.

Never content to be rank and file, they will often strive to find an area in which they can excel. Should their work go unappreciated, they may console themselves with the understanding that the ineptitude of others is to blame. Lack of skill and wisdom is why the genius of their work is not appreciated.

Pride by definition is an assumption of superiority, intellectually, financially, artistically. Their taste, skill and knowledge are in demand. Consider the following written about the social prestige and supposed artistry of the disease tuberculosis

Romancing tuberculosis was a popular pastime among writers in the eighteenth and nineteenth centuries. The disease had become Europe's number-one killer, and artists, along with the poor were falling before what John Bunyan called "the captain of all men of death." It never occurred to the scrofulous Irish living in dank Manchester cellars that glorifying death might brighten a dull career, but that's exactly what many artists did. Glassy-eyed and sad with consumption, they started the "graveyard school of poetry" and introduced Europe to the romantic mood. Graveyard writing featured weepy landscapes surreally dotted with languorous women, stone tombs and falling leaves. It also portrayed early death as both a special grace and a unique spiritual enterprise. In 1819, John Keats, an original graveyard poet, wrote that, "Youth grows pale, and spectre thin, and dies." Two years later, the twenty-six-year-old poet proved his romantic credentials by coughing himself to death.

The graveyard school drew some fantastic deductions about TB. Its members added up all the rattling "lungers" in their midst and concluded that tuberculosis had something to do with genius. The tie between intellect and TB became so strong that even healthy writers such as Alexandre Dumas pretended to look frail in order to look tragically hip. Dumas, who peopled his novels with consumptives, didn't care much for the fad but knew "it was the fashion to suffer from the lungs" and "to spit blood after each emotion that was at all sensational" Edmond and Jules de Goncourt, popular French social critics, even advised Victor Hugo to abandon his good health if he wanted to be "a greater poet". The two brothers argued that a writer needed to experience crucifixion by consumption in order to "render the delicacies, the exquisite melancholies, and rare and delicious phantasies, of the vibrant cord of the heart and soul".

In this unhealthy critical environment, peer pressure among artists to get sick or die from TB was intense. In the 1800s, most writers or composers of any merit seemed to be coughing their way to fame and an early grave. Frederick Chopin had to fight off chills and coughing fits in order to finish composing the Preludes. When tuberculosis didn't consume all of Robert Louis Stevenson's energy, he wrote The Strange Case of Dr Jekyll and Mr Hyde. The list of nineteenth-century artistic types with TB is almost as long as Toronto's phone book.

FLIRTATION AND STIMULATION

Green is the most stimuli-sensitive of all the miasms. Sex is an area where their need for stimulation can exceed the ability to deliver. The search for something new, exciting and continually different, all done with style and flair can be an unrewarding one. Frequently their partners can be at a loss to know how to behave next, as green are liable to change their minds about a fantasy at a faster rate than it takes their partners to come to terms with. The actual physical contact is, for some, a mere backdrop to the fantasy going on in their heads. A constantly creative mind combined with a strong reliance on outside stimulation, places some greens in a very dependent position. Sex, due to an inability to satisfy their creativity, can become a problem area, leaving many unfulfilled and dissatisfied.

Flirtation may become an area that green finds more stimulating than the sex or relationship that springs from it. Flirtation is about potential – any outcome is possible, it creates a question mark rather than a full stop and potential is more exciting than the result. Like mystery itself, it is the not knowing that is the most thrilling to green.

MIND; LASCIVIOUSNESS, lustfulness.

MIND; LEWDNESS, obscene.

MIND; TIMIDITY; bashful.

MIND; DREAMS; prude, being.

SENSITIVITY AND DEPENDENCE

Dependent on the help and support given by those around them, some are at a level where they cannot cope on their own. This is in harmony with their tendency to be more than adequate in one area but relatively incompetent in others. This shortfall is commonly made up by their partner or other family members. This comes in all sorts of forms, from a person who is academically or creatively brilliant but has never bothered to learn how to pay a bill, to people who could build a palace out of the scraps lying around the yard, but become emotional wrecks if left alone. Others may be a wiz around the house making their own clothes and everything tasteful but are virtually like a dependent child in all other aspects, needing to receive constant supervision and reassurance for everything they do. Whatever the situation, they are more than happy to hand over responsibility and be looked after.

Green is the only miasm so reliant on external stimuli as their prime motivator. Inspiration, stimulation, encouragement and incentive all must be drawn from outside sources; this makes them reactive rather than proactive. Weather changes or mood changes, green is sensitive to them all. Noise, appearance, odours, taste, the super-sensitive green is tuned into all stimuli. Their reputation for refinement and their artistic eye for the beautiful and pleasing, shared with their disgust for the vulgar, ugly, coarse and abrasive, can make them seem pompous and pretentious, but this may not be so. Rather than displaying their culture, sophistication and finesse, green may be reacting to their instinctive revulsion to the harsh.

GENERALITIES; WEATHER; change of; agg.

MIND; IMPRESSIONABLE, susceptible.

MIND; SENSITIVE, oversensitive.

SPITEFUL

In green it appears as if millions of years of evolution have come together to create the ultimate critic, they do it naturally and easily. Constantly evaluating, examining and comparing they appraise and assess everything. They place in hierarchies and analyse. They are judges, inspectors and evaluators by nature, making great reporters and columnists. This can also mean that during an argument they know how to dig out the deepest to hurt. Green has an acid tongue and, if pushed too far, is not afraid to use it.

This type of person is not going to give an inch, they know what you value and how to get at it. Some greens would never apply such tactics, in fact a fight of any kind is to be avoided at any cost – they will submit rather than confront, but even here some are just employing passive aggression rather than being forthright. This domesticated green gives their power to another because they live in fear, unable to trust their capabilities to look after themselves; they are willing to swap independence for security. They will create whatever you are looking for in a partner, and in a home. They will give loyalty and support, all they ask in exchange is to be taken care of and sheltered – this means constant reassurance and maintenance of the status quo. They will maniacally nag or cry if this equilibrium is disturbed until they get their way.

MIND; CONTRARY; spiteful, just to be.

MIND; BREAK things, desire to; possession, parents' most prized.

MIND; MILDNESS.

SUMMARY

Green is the most difficult miasm to define as it has the two extremes; even brown has a miasm in between to act as a moderator. There are, however, some constants like dependence. This is their most common theme, no matter how gruff or refined, many still need someone around them to help as a support and guide. Next is the perfection of their creations, and finally there exists in many an absolute way of thinking, definite constructs of which most will find it impossible to extend beyond. This is an extension of the specialist theory. This is a way of thinking that makes each either mechanical, abstract or academic but rarely a combination.

CASE 1 – Mr T aged fifty-five

Presented with a history of a detached retina and a recent diagnosis of acute angle glaucoma. Like anyone with this condition Mr T lives with the concern that he may go blind should certain symptoms occur and he does not get to a hospital in time.

He has a history of measles and whooping cough as a child as well as rubella and chicken pox.

When he was five he had his adenoids removed due to consistent nose bleeds.

At twenty-nine he had a testicle removed as it had turned gangrenous. He also has two cysts on the other testicle which had been surgically

removed at an earlier time only to grow back again. At this point they are causing him no pain and he assures me that his doctor is keeping a close eye on the problem.

He was also diagnosed with a poly-cystic right kidney, which was not removed; no one knows for certain what percentage of function exists in that kidney. There is a family history of kidney disease, his father dying of kidney failure at forty-seven.

Nine years ago, he had part of his thyroid removed and is currently on thyroxine.

He has constant sciatic pain which can occasionally go into spasms so severe that he will pass out.

He suffers from "chronic lack of sleep" and as a consequence is always tired.

He has great difficulty getting to sleep and will wake two or three times a night, sometimes up to a half an hour at a time. He could not state whether he would wake at a precise or consistent time.

He gets a type of dull headache just before an electrical storm.

He has no energy and his doctor had diagnosed him as having

chronic fatigue syndrome. This and his "sleeping disorder" are the complaints he wants addressed. All other complaints are being taking care of by his specialist.

He feels overburdened. He works too hard. He is an electrician who has his own business and has had for the past twenty-five years.

He believes his sufferings come from having to bear the heavy burdens of responsibility for too long.

He believes that he carries the burden for everybody.

He will go momentarily blind sometimes for two to three hours if exposed to bright light for too long.

He does not like spring because the season is too changeable.

He gets bored very quickly and is generally busy with ten things on the go at once.

He describes himself as a black or white person. He can go to extremes in things, rarely does he take the middle ground.

He believes that all his symptoms are telling him to finally unburden himself of the responsibility of the business.

He wants to retire next year. He wanted to retire ten years ago but still believes he needs a little longer to get himself into a financial position where he can finally relax.

He craves coca-cola and is drinking it constantly; he has an aversion to diet coke as it "lacks the necessary punch."

He eats lollies constantly.

He has regular Vitamin B-12 and Vitamin C injections for his energy levels and immune system. He needs these weekly as without them his energy goes down to zero and he will have one long continuous cold.

His hobbies include reading and watching TV; he loves listening to music. His absolute favourite is Mozart.

He likes to watch football on television but will never go to an actual game as the noise gives him a headache. He also does not like to mingle with the type of crowd that usually attends a "footy" game as they are too rough and overbearing.

He regards himself as a sensitive person, he is very reactive to stress. He loves art and architecture.

The rubrics chosen for the case were

VISION; LOSS of vision, blindness; light, by; agg.

GENERALITIES; WEATHER; storm; agg.; approach of.

MIND; SENSITIVE, oversensitive.

GENERALITIES; FOOD and drinks; sweets; desires.

MIND; RESPONSIBILITY.

NOSE; EPISTAXSIS.

EYE; GLAUCOMA.

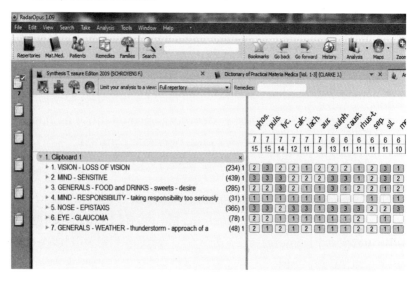

Facial features

Yellow

Freckled face

Long downward nose

Small mouth

Ears that slope backward

Blue

Deep-set eyes

Wide-set eyes

History of a now corrected underbite

His total was three blue features and four yellow features.

Mr T is green.

I did not want to extend my remedy selection below a five rubrics total so China, even though green, did not feature in the post repertorisation selection. Tuberculinum is however worth a look even though it only has four of the rubrics because it is so small. China with a more extensive proving should have featured more highly.

Phosphorus and Calc. are the remedies for consideration. Phosphorus 200 single dose was chosen.

Three weeks after the first prescription his own words were:

"Wonderful."

"I have energy to burn."

"I have started to do some exercise, I have started walking and riding my bike."

"I seem more interested in things."

"I see the sunshine more."

"I am sleeping and waking refreshed."

"I feel alive."

"I haven't had or needed my injections."

An important point with repertorisation based on a miasmatic model, is that larger rubrics can be used. It has been said by homoeopaths that larger rubrics are next to useless as they do not narrow a practitioner's field of choice. Ordinarily I would agree with this, however using this miasmatic model, our choice is automatically narrowed as approximately six-sevenths of the medicines in the repertorisation should belong to other miasmatic groups.

I next saw Mr T six months later, when after a very stressful event he was beginning to lose sleep. Phos. 200 was repeated. I see Mr T at regular three-monthly intervals because of the serious nature of his complaints, and am happy to report that he remains well.

CASE 2 – Mrs T aged seventy

Presented with eczema on her lower left leg in the college student clinic. She uses flower essences for emotional issues and is also taking prescribed medication for an overactive thyroid. The eczema commenced twenty years ago and is usually swollen and red. Over the years it has moved up her leg to her lower calf area. She uses a pressure bandage and says it usually flares up when she is stressed. The medication for her overactive thyroid has affected her taste buds, resulting in a bland taste and she is desiring sugar+++.

When asked what occurred in her life twenty years earlier she replies that she had married and the eczema had appeared during this time. She had married a man who was newly widowed and had four children including a small baby. The children she explained, were traumatized by their mother's death and she became mother to the baby but the older three did not accept her. As teenagers they would scream hate and abuse at her – there were times she wanted to kidnap the baby and leave as the situation was so emotionally unhealthy. One day after ten years her husband came to her and told her she had to leave as the children could not live with her anymore. She packed all her things and left within two hours and immediately after this her eczema became extremely bad. Privately she explained she had a breakdown.

In her day to day life she worries about money. She has many siblings and she is the only one without any children – when her siblings help and support her, the eczema lessens. In particular she worries that she will lose her house as payments are hard to keep up – she minds children but a broken ankle last year has stopped this work and she fears losing her home. When she eats a lot of sugar the eczema explodes.

During this stressful time her voice became strange – having no volume and she noticed a loss of muscle tone (during the consultation she is very softly spoken). She became very tired but couldn't sleep due to restlessness. Her previously soft fingernails became hard and brittle. "I was too tired to even be irritable".

She feels on the outer from her family with no partner and no children–sometimes she rarely sees them "it is as if I don't exist". During all the stress she cried once but never did again in public. She felt badly hurt and demoralized. Her marriage she said in her mind was for life – she had fought like fury and didn't give in – it was a shock to be told to leave.

When she was in her twenties her brother died suddenly and she got white patches in her hair overnight and experienced paralysis on her right side temporarily. She was unable to stop crying for a long time. Prior to her marriage she had migraines and during her marriage if she was screamed at she would get piercing pains < touch. She would also experience visual problems and would have to sit up and eat sweets. Her right eye is turned and she has only blurry sight in it. Since the diagnosis of the thyroid problem she has dryness in her ears – they felt brittle, dry and itchy but are not so bad now. Her nose has been blocked for the last ten years and is < lying down. Sometimes she gets cold sores in her nose and her mouth can be dry.

She has a history of regurgitation that is < cake and < oranges. Occasionally she craves wine and chocolate and she loves cheese. There is an aversion to pork. During her teens she would blackout with the pain of her periods and she didn't go through menopause at all – her periods just stopped.

In general she is < extreme heat and < extreme cold and she has cold hands. There is a history of cramps in the legs. Her sleep was very restless when the thyroid condition commenced and she would wake for two hours and then only sleep for two hours but this is better since medication. Her dreams are vivid and lively. There is some heart disease in the family but no other illnesses.

The eczema is very itchy and she wants to tear at it. When it is inflamed there is a dull pain. It is definitely < sugar and she thinks perhaps > raising the leg. It is < for lying down.

Occasionally there are feelings like electric shocks in the area.

The rubrics chosen for the case were

MIND; AILMENTS from; shock (32)

GENERALITIES; FOOD and drinks; sweets; agg. (45)

GENERALITIES; LYING; agg. (248)

SPEECH & VOICE; VOICE; weak (93)

GENERALITIES; FAINTNESS, fainting; tendency; pain, from (54)

SKIN; ERUPTIONS; eczema (177)

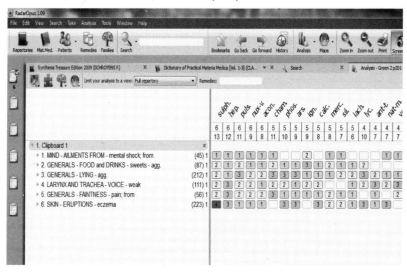

Facial features

Yellow

Two lines between eyes

Multiple lines on cheeks

Nose downturned

Smile compact

Lips thin

Forehead sloped

Downturned eyes

Red

Bridge full

Blue

Hairline high

Asymmetry – eyes, nose

Lines down from mouth Lines down from nose

Overbite

Ears large

The total of seven yellow features and six blue features shows the tubercular or green miasm.

REMEDIES

Both Hep Sulph. and Aconite were of strong consideration with Phos and Calc C. being of interest (all green remedies). Hep Sulph. read well in the materia medica (Vermuelen) and was given in 30C potency daily but with no result.

One month later Aconite 200 single dose was given. Six weeks later she attended the clinic and reported that her health was "120% better". The eczema was much improved and her thyroid was back to normal – a blood test had confirmed this. There was no irritation or swelling in her leg although it still felt a bit sensitive and was slightly pink. Her low voice was back to normal and her energy was so good "I am able to wash my car

– which I haven't been able to do without being exhausted for years" Her attitude is positive – "people have been flooding me with things" and she hasn't been crying on her own. Although she still has financial difficulties she is not worried and knows everything will be fine. One month further on she is still feeling "terrific and full of energy". Six months later she is contacted by phone and still remains well.

THE GENERALS OF GREEN

AGGRAVATIONS

Lifting and overstraining
Ascending
Shock
Change of weather
Loss of fluids
Fasting
Exertion
Continuous motion
Dark
Becoming cold
Noise
Thinking of complaints
Extended concentration
Stress and worry

AMELIORATIONS

Dark
Pressure
Rubbing
Touch
Gentle motion

Rapid motion
Eating
Diverting the attention
Open air

SENSATIONS
Sour
Numb
Trembling
Cold
Weak
Empty
Sluggish

REPRODUCTIVE
Lascivious fantasies with a fear to fulfil them
Desire stronger than ability
Sexual excess
Dependence on partner for stimulation.

FOOD
Indigestibles
Sweets
Spices
Fruit
Stimulants

PATHOLOGY
Profuse perspiration. Rapid emaciation. Cancer. **Polyps**. Nervous exhaustion. **R.S.I.** Headaches. Neuralgia. **Croup**. Insomnia. **Sprains and strains**. Adenoids. **Convulsions**. Spinal curvatures. **Repeated colds**. Haemorrhages. Varicose veins. Whooping cough. Tinnitus. Measles. Asthma. Repeated throat problems. **Kidney disorders**. Arthritis. Osteoporosis. Abscess. Orchitis.

CHAPTER 20

Miasmatic Themes - Cancer (Brown)

There are fewer explanations into the character of this miasm when compared to the others as, being a conglomerate, brown is capable of exhibiting any or all of the traits covered by the other miasms. In miasmatic prescribing one should always be aware that brown can resemble any theme. Only facial feature identification will determine whether your patient is yellow or brown, red or brown, purple or brown, etc. This being said there are some aspects of character that belong, not exclusively, but certainly most centrally to brown.

FEAR, ANTICIPATION AND THE NEED FOR SUPPORT

With Arsenicum as one of the brown miasm's primary flagship remedies, an understanding of the type of nervous energy displayed by this miasm is instantly recognisable. In fact only purple can equal brown in frenetic energy. Both brown and purple as a consequence tend to be the most prone to high anxiety disorders and panic attacks. Brown can be pessimistic, never trusting life to provide an adequate answer. Not leaving anything to chance, brown may try and police everything, guaranteeing that nothing goes past unnoticed. Full of restless energy, brown can be either a power house or, if turned inward, a neurotic bundle of nerves unable to relax even for a second. This is best recognised during illness where some may become hypochondriacal. Fearing both death and disease, they will demand support, unable to settle until an adequate answer to their suffering has been found. To this end brown can be a demanding patient both in time and services. Like purple, brown may play on their practitioner's humanitarian nature to understand the depth of their plight, explain why they need extra effort, only to leave your clinic for their next appointment with a different practitioner. In reference to homoeopathy brown can again rival purple with their propensity for continual self-prescription. The opposite is just as true where many will provide no self-care or support, no matter how obvious until advised to do so by someone else. This type can be so indifferent to everything around them, generally through exhaustion, that they simply accept everything that happens to them.

A sense of mania can pursue brown. So cluttered can their thoughts be they can believe they are going mad, easy to understand as they have all the miasms telling them what to do. Their mania or depression can be as strong as that of blue only with brown there is a constant need for reassurance. This is a miasm that needs support, being alone or self-supporting is a hard thing for them.

One of the most difficult concepts to bear in mind is that it can display and mimic every other miasmatic group, as it contains all those preceding it.

OBSESSIVE BEHAVIOUR AND ATTENTION TO DETAIL

Following on from the miasmatic theme presented in fear,

anticipation, and the need for support, obsessive and compulsive behaviour can be a predictable sequelae to such an anxious personality. With nervous energy to spare brown is often highly detailed to the point of fixation. Never leaving anything to chance they will focus on the smallest detail making sure every "i is dotted" and every "t is crossed".

With so much inner turmoil it is not surprising they need their external environment as ordered as possible. This excessive attention to detail is a major contributor to the Arsenicum and Carcinosin drug pictures. These characterisations give them a reputation for cleanliness and exacting behaviour. This can make them seem dictatorial and demanding to those around them, driving others to reach the same levels of competence as themselves. Fastidiousness can be a valuable asset if regulated properly, but most of the time it is not for, once again, despite all of their self-promises, they will find themselves falling into the same old patterns. Like all disease, it is easier to succumb than to transcend. This raises an important question. How can people change if a miasm has such a strong hold of them? Miasmatic prescribing does not suggest that people stay the one stable personality. Individuals constantly change aspects of their character, what is being emphasised is the importance of an environmental shift to elicit a response. Albert Einstein once stated that insanity is: "Doing the same old thing over and over again and expecting different results." A change in character is, more precisely, a different response from the same character due to a change in circumstance.

Brown can be industry's workhorse, their attention to detail and inability to rest until each task is completed makes them a dependable employee who often takes on more responsibilities than there are hours in the day. This tendency leads them into exploitation, a position they may find themselves in constantly whether at work, or in relationships, their good natures are forever being taken advantage of. Brown must be on a constant vigil to guard against this misuse of their character. Without doubt, of all of the consultations I have ever done with brown patients, this issue above all others is the most reccurring. They may be the most reliable, or the softest touch, or the best craftsman or the most cheap and dependable worker; whatever the reason others will want their services and brown cannot say no. This is their own fault, they need to be stronger and understand that they can say no and still be loved, liked or respected. But sometimes it goes further than this, where others begin to expect them to behave a certain way, such as the mother who cleans and prepares everything so no one else has to lift a finger, or the worker whose tasks are always finished on time and to perfection even though others around them are redirecting much of their workload to them, often without so much as a thank you. This is the exploitation that can await them throughout their lives if they are unwary.

Anticipating the worst, brown try and safeguard every event before it occurs. Left to chance anything is possible so, as a consequence, they will take control of the reins and direct proceedings. To some this will be interpreted as interference or control, and many from this miasm will indeed cross this line, but most will not see their behaviour as such. Through their eyes they are offering help and delivering an attention to detail that was sorely lacking previously. Misunderstanding others' aversion to too much concentration on loose ends, they feel their efforts are unappreciated as the recipient may seem to be more annoyed than grateful. Failing to grasp they are feeling bogged down in detail, brown may misjudge the anxiousness of others to get on with the job. Brown are often accused of missing the big picture.

MIND; COMPULSIVE disorders.

MIND; TRIFLES; important, seem.

MIND; ANXIETY; anticipating.

MIND; AVARICE.

MIND; CONTRADICTION; intolerant of.

MIND; FASTIDIOUS.

ENEMIES AND PARANOIA

Perhaps as an extension of the red side of their character, brown can suffer from the same sense of persecution as the deepest red remedy. Brown is extremely protective of what they have, whether it's possessions, ideas or people, all things become a focus of their obsessive tendency. Their paranoia can range from believing others are trying to take things from them, to believing that people are out to harm them either physically or professionally. Physically others are attacking them, making them suffer or deliberately letting them suffer. Professionally they are spreading lies and gossip about them, deliberately running their good name down in front of potentially important people, trying to get out of work and still be a hero at the same time. To a brown in this state, everyone is up to some kind of mischief. People are always trying to manipulate them or the system, in order to ruin others and personally profit. The world is full of leeches that will suck out all the life blood they can get if not stopped, brown are the self-appointed watchdogs against these people. These people are using the system to their own ends, deceiving others in the process by making them think they are contributing rather than exploiting. For brown, exploitation is a prime energy pattern, whether, as previously stated, it is they that are exploited, or it is stopping others from exploiting them, their profession, hobby or system. This combined with an inherited sense of justice makes brown the ultimate policeman.

MIND; DELUSIONS, imaginations; injury; receive, will.

MIND; DELUSIONS, imaginations; thieves, robbers, sees.

MIND; DELUSIONS, imaginations; thieves, robbers, sees; house, in.

MIND; DELUSIONS, imaginations; watched, that she is being.

DESIRE TO SELF-NURTURE, PURITY AND DEFILEMENT

Brown has a strong subconscious desire to nurture their souls and find some peace. Most miasms will take time out and say enough is enough. Most have a cut-off point where the most self-nurturing and protective thing to do is say no. Most from this miasm have a cut-off point, but some have a far more extended cut-off point than what is responsible. Saying no, in any of its forms, work, home, social engagements, can be something they find difficult to do. This shows poor self-worth, a feeling they cannot demand anything for themselves. Brown is someone who does not contribute except in a way they think others want them to. Brown tries to be all things to all people. Some, having no identity of their own, may borrow an image they feel is the nicest and most pleasing to as broad a group as possible. This is where many of their long-term problems begin, for their identity can be replaced by a role. If there is one word that describes a brown in this position – it is *lost*

Being natural givers, some with a more well-balanced attitude will find time to regenerate. Having an outlet is vital for the give and take of energy. Many find their best form of self-nurture and expression is in one of the arts. Whether in painting, literature or the theatre, many find a valuable safety valve in art. Much is made of green's artistic bent, but in reality I have seen more brown artists than green.

THE SAME MISTAKES

Learning not to make the same mistakes with the same people, or at least the same sort of people, is one of this miasms life challenges. The "once bitten" motto is not something brown adopt naturally. This can be seen in Foubister's description of Carcinosin. He describes an immune system failing in its task of learning and identification and, as a consequence, childhood illnesses are repeated two, even three times. They may suffer constantly from a recurring illness or, just as frequently, be left with the continuing effects of a disease long after the actual contagion has spent its force – chronic fatigue syndrome after glandular fever or influenza is a prime example of this.

Mentally, they can be the type who consistently believes, for whatever reason, the false promises of people who have repeatedly let them down in the past, always coming back for more and setting themselves up for further violence and exploitation. An extension of this, more recognised by those around them than in themselves, is their general naivety. Seen in their continuous belief in false promises, their dedication can be to the point of gullibility. Their acceptance places them in predicaments few others would tolerate. Indeed, their trusting nature is often viewed by others as a blatant lack of caution. This naivety can also include an inability to grasp subtleties.

Many times it will be brown that says something they shouldn't without intent or malice, only to find that people are angry with them for their lack of tact and understanding. At other times they will be last to grasp the fact that a joke has passed its use-by date, continuing with it they will be the only one not to get a laugh.

SPIRITUALITY AND THE SEARCH FOR IDENTITY

Seen often in Carcinosin and even more so in Silica is the search for meaning and spirituality. More than any other miasm, it is brown that is the guru or sect worshipper. Like red with love, brown are looking for someone or something to which they can devote themselves. According to the mechanics of devotion, one must bestow all their faith and trust into the hands of another. This ability to entirely give themselves over, as a sacrifice, is a trait that comes too easily for their own good, once again the conditions for exploitation are in place. Brown has a strange relationship with power; like purple, it can be dictatorial or completely submissive. However dictatorial browns are far less likely to take advantage of those in submissive positions than purple.

Having every miasmatic influence, there is internal confusion; frequently in brown it manifests as an identity vacuum. Desperate to find some distinctiveness, they resort to any means that help give an understanding of who they are. There is a strong wish to be identifiable and recognisable, someone unique and separate from others. Personality projection can take the form of a cause, where they adopt an ethic or lifestyle around a particular belief, their whole personality becoming an extension of how they believe a greenie or an artist should behave. Often it is a spiritual path and, true to form, their compliance will be as strict as the best ascetic and always in character.

An inherent drive for spiritual understanding, combined with an ability to comprehend all aspects of human nature, helps brown achieve a spiritual depth and a level of compassionate understanding few from any another miasm can attain. Brown can be truly humble, kind and giving. I would not be surprised to find that many of the great spiritual teachers were brown.

SO PERFECT YET SO DESTRUCTIVE

Always smiling is a good description of this type of brown. Less fastidious and more social, they are truly one of God's gifts. On the positive side they are one of the most well-respected and loved of all people. They are caring and nurturing. There is not a single thing they would not do for somebody, they are the complete carer, always on call and never overburdened. This type is the person that will donate their life to sponsoring children, saving animals, the local football club, the local school and so forth. Whatever is the hobby of their partners or children (usually children as they require more nurturing and that is what brown is looking for) is now, by association, their passion too. To some this devotion is simply being supportive, but miasmatically it still shows the tendency towards personality adoption and self-sacrifice.

If this behaviour pattern stops at this level and does not progress any further then, provided they live in an environment where they are free to express themselves, many will go on to live a wonderful life, die in their nineties and have hundreds of people at their funeral. But should they completely lose themselves in a role, believing their whole purpose is to serve, the consequences can be very dire indeed. "The good die young" the saying states, and this good someone may very well be brown. Sacrifice is regarded as an honourable thing, the whole Christian tradition is modelled on it, but the gains have to be worthwhile, otherwise it is futile. While brown value others, they also need to be valued in the right and most respectful way. They must also value themselves. Like every colour, brown build for themselves a miasmatic catch 22. In order to have self-value, they must be valued by others. They accomplish this by their instinctual nature to give, but some over-give which can lead to their being exploited. They can find themselves surrounded by disrespectful and unquenchable demands. They in turn respond by doing more, and so it continues, until eventually they are lost in a sea of selfishness and have simply become a role, losing all the value they were aspiring to attain.

Too many times have I have heard a confession of "I am loved but I am not respected". "How could they respect me?" was the reply one brown patient stated, "They don't even know me and I've been living in the house for thirty years". Things don't have to be this way, perhaps if this patient had been a little more forceful rather than so accepting, things may have been different, but that is not how this miasm operates.

With all this giving, it comes as no surprise to find they are tired all the time. Fatigue is the most common single complaint suffered by this miasm and may extend into their facial appearance. This statement is hard to explain as it is a quality rather than a distinctive feature, but a drawn and tired "feel" often surrounds them. It could not be otherwise, in brown: all their energy is going out and very little is coming back in; this continuous output eats into their reserves, causing problems, especially with the brown type who are "born tired".

Striving for perfection is another aspect of this miasm, whether in obvious ways such as engineering, art or sport, or being the perfect student or the perfect human being. What brown really desires is to relax, to let someone else clean up the mess; they want others to show them how important they are, to have others prove to them that they are loved and wanted. Brown must be careful, in their desperation to be loved and treated nicely some are willing to do almost anything, and this may cost them dearly. They have inherited a fear of being alone but many end up alone anyway, it's just that they spend their loneliness surrounded by people. These browns fear to open up and tell others how they feel because they wouldn't want to offend anybody.

At this point it is important to stress that all are acting in accordance with their predisposition. They cannot change their personality any more than others can. To tell a sweet brown to stop being generous is like telling your heart not to beat.

MIND; SMILING.

MIND; CARRIED; desires to be; fondled, and.

MIND; FEAR; approaching; others, of.

MIND; FEAR; alone, of.

MIND; DREAMS; dirt; linen, dirty.

DREAMS; urinating, of; decent manner, in, when he is wetting the bed at night.

SUPPRESSION

For this miasm, illness can be a respectable and legitimate

excuse for non-continuance. Suicide is a strong tendency that runs through brown but, unlike blue, it is best understood as a subconscious desire to escape from a relentless situation or problem, rarely is it a consciously acknowledged suicidal thought. Clarke says:

I have met with a suicidal tendency in several cancer patients, so that the cancer nosodes may be appropriate in many mental cases, especially where the heredity points that way.

As an example, it is well known that Carcinosin is a good remedy for chronic fatigue syndrome; it is no coincidence that so many people who get CFS do so in highly stressful and pivotal moments. The straight "A" student who gets it in their last year of high school, or the athlete who is "struck down" by chronic fatigue at the peak of their career, are an all too familiar story. True to their nature many will battle on regardless. Cancer for is the same excuse, with a different disease manifestation. Obviously the seriousness of the disease will correspond to the seriousness of the problem. For some it is a way of unburdening a long borne weight. In this way browns gain a legitimate way to finally be nurtured and appreciated; dissolving their responsibilities, the carer finally becomes the cared for.

"Never well since mononucleosis".

BROWN CASES

CASE 1 – Mr B R aged sixty-two

Mr B R came to the clinic suffering with repeated herpes virus that was worse each spring. The herpetic eruption is worse on the left arm and on the left side of the penis. Normally he is very active but every time he gets a virus he is depressed because of his lack of energy. On occasions he also suffered colds that would settle in his nose and throat. When sick he gets hot flushes followed by chills. His skin is very sensitive to the touch. Sometimes he takes Aconite when sick as he feels restless and he believes it helps him. He can get flushes every half an hour when sick and also gets hives on some occasions. He describes himself as outgoing and busy. He is reluctant to talk much more about himself. He was given Lach. 1M as this was an early test case and facial features were not taking precedence over presenting symptomology. It had no result. He returned six months later feeling very unwell especially since being overseas in a hot climate. During the journey he had a lot of travel sickness with dizziness. On further questioning he admits to being fearful of accidents and that he suffers heartburn when stressed or eating fatty food. His sleeping is poor and he often wakes at 4 a.m. He has recurring dreams about being naked or needing to use the toilet at inappropriate times. He says he suffers muscle twitches in his legs during the night along with cramps in the lower limbs. He has had two outbreaks of herpetic eruptions in the last six months.

The rubrics chosen for his case were:

MIND; FEAR; accidents, of.

MIND; DREAMS; nakedness, about.

GENERALITIES; SIDE; left.

GENERALITIES; WARMTH; agg.

WAKING; midnight; after four a.m.

EXTREMITIES; TWITCHING; night.

EXTREMITIES; CRAMPS; lower limbs.

SKIN; ERUPTIONS; herpetic.

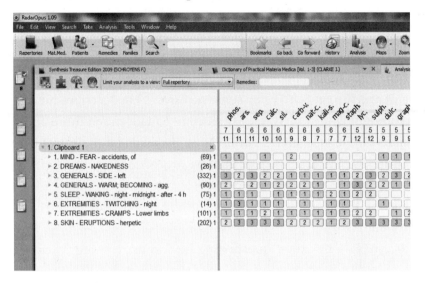

Facial features

Yellow

Eyes close set

Eyes down-turned

Forehead – worry lines

Nose – bump on profile

Red

Lips full

Teeth even

Full bridge of nose

Blue

Eyes deep set

Asymmetry nose/eyes

Deep lines from corners of nose to corners of mouth

Lower lip protrudes on profile

Mr B R is brown as he has an equal mix of all three primary miasms.

Arsenicum 1M single dose was given. One month later he returned and is feeling much better. His sleep has improved and he isn't waking or getting cramps or twitches. The eruption on his arm and penis have vanished and he feels generally more relaxed and energetic. Six months later he remains well. The following spring the eruption threatened to recur. Arsenicum 1M was repeated.

No recurrence.

CASE 2 – Mr S M aged forty-nine

Mr S M aged forty-nine presents with digestive troubles and a diagnosis of candida. He suffers with dizziness and an inability to eat that is much worse when he becomes cold. His tongue is coated white and his teeth leave an imprint. He feels worse for eating fatty food, sweets and bread and has an aversion to alcohol. He is married with three children and likes to work alone. This is possible as the business he works for allows him the freedom to work as he chooses – he is an architect. His greatest dislike is dealing with competitive people and he hates fights or confrontation. By nature he is a peaceful person and spent much of his younger years visiting ashrams in India to meditate. He loves eastern philosophy. His father was aggressive and unpredictable. As well as digestive troubles he gets mouth ulcers especially on the gums and pimples around his nose, mouth and shoulders. He says, "I have been trying to work out my identity most of my life" and that he has "a poor sense of self-worth". Relationships must be truthful and sincere and he describes his wife as fulfilling his needs. When asked about fears he says he fears losing control in a conflict, as years of anger may come out.

The rubrics chosen for his case were

MIND; RELIGIOUS affections.

GENERALITIES; COLD; becoming; agg.

GENERALITIES; FOOD and drinks; fats and rich food; agg.

MIND; CONFIDENCE; want of self.

MOUTH; COATED; tongue, white.

MOUTH; ULCERS; gums.

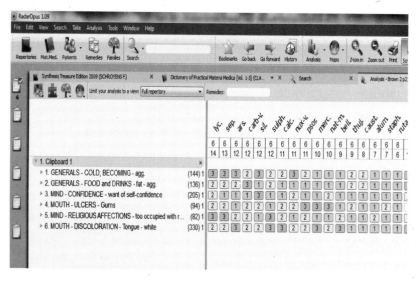

Facial features

Yellow

Eyes down-turned

Forehead – worry lines

Nose – bump on profile

Forehead sloped back

Red

Mouth wide

Ears pinned back at top

Nose wide

Single line between eyes

Blue

Eyes and mouth asymmetrical

Vertical lines in cheeks

Chin defined, jutting appearance

Mr S M belongs to the brown miasm. Silica and Arsenicum are our choices. Silica is chosen due to his introverted nature and aversion to confrontation. Silica 1M single dose. One month later his improvement is considerable. He has no stomach troubles at all and the dizziness has gone. Although still weak due to previous loss of weight, his eating patterns are now back to normal and his weight is beginning to increase. His mouth ulcers have cleared and his general energy is good. Three months later he began to slip back and his nausea and aggravation from the cold were returning. Silica 1M was repeated and all symptoms cleared quickly. Six months later he was back to full weight and remains well.

THE GENERALS OF BROWN

AGGRAVATIONS

Exertion

Old age

Touch

Injuries and blows

Sea

Loss of fluids

Lifting

Menses

Coition

AMELIORATIONS

Warmth

Sleep

Motion

Fasting

Knee-chest position

Pressure

Sitting

SENSATIONS

Weak

Worn out

Tired

Burning

Violent

Cold

Sticking

Stabbing

Burning

Numb

Knotty

Gone

Twitching

Creeping

Peppery

Cold

Violent

Quivering

REPRODUCTIVE

Cracked nipples

Inverted nipples

Coition aggravates

Sterility

Aversion to coition

Lack of desire

False pregnancy

Bleeding either during or after sex

Painful coition

FOOD

Desire for and aggravation from fats and rich food

Butter

Salt

Aggravation from alcohol

Aversion to sweets

Loathing of food

Desires sour

Aggravation from hot drinks

PATHOLOGY

Fainting. **Cancer. Tumours.** Polyps. Glandular affections. Spine. **Diabetes. Gangrene** and other sceptic conditions. Ulcers. Acne. **Rheumatoid arthritis. Lupus.** Keloid scaring. **CFS.** Problems with the hair and nails. **Glandular fever.** Severe influenza. **Pneumonia.** Repeated high fevers. Emphysema. Hepatitis. **Chronic post-nasal infections.** Thalassemia. **Insomnia.** Fissures. Spina bifida.

PART THREE
FACIAL FEATURES

CHAPTER 21

How to Interpret Facial Features

A patient can be observed in two ways. The first is by direct observation in the clinic. This will provide some feature recognition but more importantly gives quality and essence. The second is by taking photos. Photos give facial feature clarity and an opportunity to scrutinise the features without making the patient feel too uncomfortable. Both methods are important and provide valuable information. For example many facial lines do not show up in photos but are clearly observable in the clinic whereas photos will often show an asymmetry that is not seen by direct observation alone.

TAKING THE PHOTOS

There are six* photos that need to be taken to get all the information required.

- Full frontal of face with a relaxed (normal) expression
- Full frontal of face with hair pulled back to reveal shape of hair line
- Full frontal of face with natural smile
- Full frontal of face with broad smile to reveal teeth

- Profile of face (both sides) with hair pulled back to reveal full profile of forehead, profile of nose and position and shape of ears.

Footnote 2008 – We now recommend a total of seven photos. All the above plus a "frown" photo – which highlights lines between the eyes

Online video on how to take photos

http://www.soulandsurvival.org/content/hfa-how-take-photos

Some patients don't smile widely enough to reveal their teeth (some patients won't smile at all – even getting them to grimace will show their teeth). It is very important to analyse the teeth to get accurate information.

It is important that the patient hold their head as straight as possible otherwise a bad angle may be mistaken for asymmetry. The profile photo must also be straight to observe the forehead, bridge of nose and nose correctly. Sometimes lines in the face won't appear in the photos. This can be seen when a patient frowns and, for example, they may have one single or two double lines between the eyes. Either take a photo of the patient frowning or just make a note to be included in the chart. All photos are best taken on a high resolution digital camera for the following reasons.

- Photos are immediately downloaded to a computer so each photo can be quickly and accurately stored with the patient's case. Downloading directly to a computer also allows for zooming in on a feature for further clarity.
- Each case can be reviewed immediately to ensure greater accuracy of the facial diagnosis.

SURGERY/WIGS/TEETH

The need to be informed about any previous surgery, wigs or dental work becomes obvious. There is no use marking down a patient's nice straight teeth as red if years of dental work has been endured correcting an over-or under-bite. In a case such as this, the overbite becomes the feature to be included, not the straight teeth. Hence the teeth will be marked as blue and not red.

The same will also apply if a patient has false teeth. As an example, if they have had false teeth since their teens because their teeth turned black and corroded, then the original state of the teeth must be the indicator. Such teeth would be counted as a blue feature.

ANALYSING THE FEATURES

- Use a copy of CHART OF FEATURES to record and tally symptoms. (See page 287 and 442-443)

    - Work your way slowly through the face recording OBVIOUS features that you can recognise – follow the order of the chart.

    - Give one point for each obvious feature.

    - If the feature isn't clear or you can't read it – leave it out or put a question mark*.

    - The totality of features will give you the final analysis – usually between eight and twenty features (less in young children and more in older people).

    - Once complete, tally the points for each of the primary miasms (yellow, red and blue).

    - Where one miasm is TWO POINTS OR MORE ahead of

the others it will be the dominant miasm.

- Where two miasms are WITHIN ONE POINT of one another the patient will be one of the double complex miasms (orange, purple or green).

- Where all three miasms are WITHIN ONE POINT of one another the patient will be brown.

> *Footnote 2008 – If a feature is not clear but could be included note it with a question mark. Using question marks allows for a totality overview which can help when deciding what the total miasmatic dominance of the case will be.

ASSESSING THE FEATURES

It has been shown via experience that any colour that is a clear *two features or more* ahead of its next nearest miasm will be the dominant miasm from which the remedy must be chosen. This figure was arrived at through numerous clinical cases. A miasm that is lower in its presence by two or more features will not exert enough influence on the patient and is to be disregarded.

For example:

YELLOW	RED	BLUE
7	5	2

= YELLOW

Yellow holds such dominance that the other two miasms cannot exert control.

YELLOW	RED	BLUE
7	6	4

= ORANGE

In this patient there is only one feature difference between yellow and red. Blue on the other hand being more than two features behind the dominant miasm (yellow with seven features) cannot hold influence to the same degree as the yellow or red features. The patient will fit the orange miasm.

YELLOW	RED	BLUE
4	7	6

= PURPLE

YELLOW	RED	BLUE
7	4	6

= GREEN

YELLOW	RED	BLUE
7	5	4

= YELLOW

YELLOW	RED	BLUE
5	4	4

= BROWN

YELLOW	RED	BLUE
3	4	2

= ORANGE

This understanding has been arrived at via clinical experience. Many cases of trial and error have shown the accuracy of this decision. No system is foolproof and sometimes features that were obvious in the first analysis are not so obvious in the second. Sometimes it may take a few tries to get the miasm right. This is the human error that exists in every system and must be accepted as such to avoid unnecessary self-criticism. Don't force the analysis. Let it be delivered to you – if you cannot make sense of a feature leave it and move on to the next. Mistakes will be made and sometimes features will be confusing but what aspects of homoeopathy are not? Enjoy this method and incorporate it into your practice no matter which other method you practise. You will find it a helpful and enthralling adjunct to your remedy choices.

NOTE – When counting asymmetry as a BLUE feature it must occur in TWO places in the face (e.g nose and eyes, or eyes and mouth) to be given ONE point.

Note on Chart

This chart has been added from the Homœopathic Facial Analysis book (published 2006) and is an updated version of the original chart in Appearance and Circumstance. Some of the features in Appearance and Circumstance (2003) have been upgraded and either renamed or dropped due to their rarity or difficulty in definition.

CHART OF FEATURES

TYPE	YELLOW	RED	BLUE
Hairline	Widows peak M shape	Straight Low Crowded	High/Balding Crooked
Forehead	Sloped (straight 12° or greater)	Straight (vertical to 11°) Brow strong	Curved Indented
Bridge		Full/Straight	Indented
Eyes	Down turned Close-set Small Full lids	Large Exopthalmic	Upturned Wide-set Deep-set Recessed lids Eye indents - new feature see HFA online course
Nose	Down turned Curved Bump	Wide Ball Cleft+	
Cheeks			Bones strong Sunken under
Mouth	Small	Wide	
Lips	Thin	Full	Under-lip (profile)
Smile	Compact	Full Large Gums show	
Teeth	Front two prominent	Even Gaps (between front teeth or multiple)	Crooked Crossed over front two* Sharp/pointed Cupped Overbite Under bite Inward
Chin	Sloped back	Ball Cleft	Defined Pointed
Ears	High Low Sloped	Turned out Turned in	Large Small
Lines	Forehead Eyes – below Eyes – two between Cheeks – multiple fine	Eyes – one between Mouth – around	Bridge – horizontal Cheeks – dimples/lines Nose – down from Mouth – down from Beside eyes-indents
Asymmetry			Two places on face = 1 point
Skin	Freckles		

+ No example in book

* Classified incorrectly as yellow in *Appearance and Circumstance* – since confirmed as blue

HFA REMEDY CLASSIFICATION

Confirmed remedies

Yellow	Red	Blue	Orange	Purple	Green	Brown
Allium Cepa	Agaricus M	Aurum Met	Chamomilla	Anacardium	Aconite	Alumina
Bryonia Alb	Ant Crud	Baryta Carb	Ferrum Met	Belladonna	Bacillinum	Arg Nit
Carbo Veg	Apis	Cantharis V	Ignatia	Hyoscyamus	Calc Carb	Ars Alb
Chelidonium	Arnica	Conium	Nat Mur	Lachesis	Calc Phos	Carcinosin
Graphites	Cannabis Ind	Mercury	Nux Vom	Nit Ac	China	Causticum
Kali Carb	Dulcamara	Mezerium		Platina	Hep Sulph	Mag Carb
Lycopodium	Medorrhinum	Plumbum		Staphysagria	Phosphorus	Mag Mur
Opium	Rhus Tox	Syphilinum		Stramonium	Sanguinaria	Nat Carb
Petroleum	Sepia			Veratrum Alb	Tuberculinum	Phos Ac
Psorinum	Tarentula H					Silica
Pulsatilla	Thuja					Zinc
Sulphur						

Under testing

Yellow	Red	Blue	Orange	Purple	Green	Brown
Ammon Carb	Bellis Per	Aethusia Cyn	Aloe Soc	Ant Tart	Asarum Eur	Coffea Cruda
Berberis V	Cannabis S	Agnus Cast	Cactus	Cenchris	Calc Fl	Hydrastis
Haliae-ic	Cimicifuga	Ambra Gris	Calendula	Cocculus Ind	Calc Sul	Selenium
Lilium Tig	Formica	Borax	Carbon Sul	Colchicum	Gelsemium	Tabacum
Podophyllum	Hydrogen	Carb An	Colocynthis	Crot Horr	Kali Bich	
Ranunculus B	Ipec	Cicuta Vir	Nat Sulph	Cyclamen	Kali Phos	
Spongia	Sabina	Eup Perf	Stannum	Lac Can	Nat Phos	
	Variolinum	Fl Ac	Sul Ac	Lyssin	Ruta Grav	
		Iodum		Naja		
		Kali Iod		Vipera		
		Phytolacca				

Latest HFA remedy information
https://www.vcch.org/remedies.html

CHAPTER 22

How to Read a Face

The first thing to understand about facial analysis is that it relates to shape and structure, not looks or beauty. It examines individual features not overall appearance.

Everything regarding the application of miasmatic facial analysis, centres on measuring the impact of psora, syphilis and sycosis. Facial analysis comes from homoeopathy and is designed specifically for homoeopathic use. Its intent is homoeopathic and its application is homoeopathic.

Miasms affect facial features in three distinct ways

1. Small, thin and sloped (psora - yellow)

2. Large, full and straight (sycosis - red)

3. Inward, sharp and asymmetrical (syphilis - blue)

The best way of analysing a face is to divide a page into three sections headed yellow, red and blue.

YELLOW	RED	BLUE
Widows peak	Full bridge	Recessed lids
Curved nose	Large eyes	Asymmetry
Sloping chin	Full lips	Dimples
	Full smile	

These yellow, red and blue columns represent psora, sycosis and syphilis, the three chronic miasms of Hahnemann. All chronic disease, regardless of pathological name, is either a product of one of these miasms or a combination of them.

Three pillars form the foundation of homoeopathy

1. The law of similars

2. The totality of symptoms

3. The infinitesimal dose

At the heart of all homoeopathy lies the law of similars. A natural law that is incontrovertible and inflexible. Attraction and repulsion is the fundamental principle that binds the universe together. It is the heart of homoeopathic theory and the rock upon which all else is built. The totality of symptoms is our key to the similimum and the infinitesimal dose is how we apply it, but the similimum is always the objective.

In chronic disease, two similar diseases cannot live in the same body at the same time, because two similar diseases – of equal strength – 'annihilate' one another (Aphorism 43 & 45) leaving the patient cured. Whereas, two dissimilar diseases never cure, they either join to form a 'complex disease' (Aphorism 40) or else the stronger will repel the weaker (Aphorism 36). Hahnemann also talked of one dissimilar disease suspending the other until the stronger has run its course, then, the old – weaker disease – will return (Aphorism 38) but in this case the stronger dissimilar disease is acute, not chronic.

If we do not understand these laws, we fail to utilise homoeopathy and run the risk of running off on a tangent. Each primary miasm is a dissimilar disease. Pathology in all of its forms and titles is just an example of these dissimilar diseases at work. The true diagnosis is always psora, sycosis or syphilis. Psora is reactive and hypoproductive, sycosis is inflammatory and hyper-productive and syphilis is submissive and destructive. All the diseases known to humankind affect the body in either one of these three ways or in a 'complex' combination of them.

Yellow, red and blue are the only miasms considered when examining a face because they are the only true chronic dissimilar diseases. Facial features are rated yellow, red and blue to represent each miasm.

CATEGORISING FEATURES

If a patient's eyelids are recessed, they feature as one blue point; this feature is noted in the blue column.

YELLOW	RED	BLUE
		Recessed eyelids

However if a patient's eyes are exophthalmic they are red, and this feature is placed in the red column.

YELLOW	RED	BLUE
	Exophthalmic eyes	

In this method, facial features are analysed and rated according to shape and appearance. Classifying facial features by the process of small, thin and sloping for yellow, large, round or straight for red and asymmetrical, inward or pointed for blue is generally accurate although there are some exceptions to the rule.

When analysing facial features do not to be in a hurry and do not feel you have to classify every feature. Take your time to compare each feature and examine it in relation to the other features on the face. This is the process of miasmatic classification.

Small eyes for example, may not be small because they are 'X' amount of centi-metres wide, but because they are small by comparison to the patient's other facial features. In this sense, a person may have small eyes because;

1. They are anatomically smaller than average
2. They are small compared to the size of the other facial features

It is important to take note of facial features without being obtrusive. Digital cameras give valuable insight, but never downplay the importance of information gathered during the one on one consultation. For example, when a person smiles or laughs during the consultation their smile may be compact. However, a photograph may not show the compact nature of this smile because the smile is not a natural one, it is a camera smile and they are rarely as broad as when a person smiles with delight.

Facial lines are another area where a one on one evaluation is important, because the camera does not show the depth of facial lines and sometimes will not show any lines at all. It is important to take notice of these features during the consultation. Patients go through a gamut of emotions during a consultation and their face will pull numerous expressions. We need to be observant to catch all these expressions so we can take note of their lines, curves and facial idiosyncrasies to fill in the gaps the camera leaves behind.

A digital camera supplies information difficult to obtain with the naked eye without highly obtrusive examination. Asymmetry is an example of this. Occasionally the naked eye may pick up the subtlety of ears not aligned or eyes of a slightly different shape, a nose gently curved or one side of the face that is higher than the other. Generally, however, it is the camera that discovers these details.

Digital photographs allow for close up examination while the naked eye reveals subtlety, expression and depth. Both the camera and good observational skills are required if clinical practice is to be successful using this method.

Assessing facial features is not fool proof and much depends on the eye and mind of the assessor. Some practitioners examine in excruciating detail, every feature and spot. Personally, I believe this is unnecessary and often such attention to detail is more of a hindrance than a help.

RUBRICS AND FACIAL ANALYSIS

Facial analysis is like repertorising. At the end of a typical constitutional consultation, the practitioner has one to ten pages of information. From this information, they choose four to eight rubrics on average. Rubrics are a summary of the important aspects of the case. Too many rubrics will discriminate against small to medium sized remedies, while too few rubrics are not enough for totality. From the repertorisation, we select a remedy and give it to the patient.

Remember, for good consistent results, rubrics must be obvious and poignant. Life is activity and motion is observable. To understand where a person's priority lies, observe what they make time to do. No one has time to accomplish all the things they want to do, so we prioritise. What we make time for represents who we are and what we value. People always find time to do what they really want to do. As the old saying goes – actions speak louder than words.

Repertorisation is a summary of the important aspects in a case it is not every spoken word. In the same way, facial analysis is about the obvious – not the barely visible or unseen. Concentrate on what is real, not on what is speculative. If you have to squint, hunt, guess, or deliberate for too long a period, then you need to question how relevant that feature truly is. At the same time, flippancy is never a way to accomplish anything.

Facial features display the dominant miasm and its influence on the system, and this dominant miasms presence will not be delicate; the dominant miasm dictates all internal and external affairs, it has full authority and power – it is *not* subtle.

THE PRACTICAL ASPECT OF FACIAL ANALYSIS

Some faces are very clear and the miasm is obvious. Others are more subtle and each feature must be checked carefully. There is an error margin of only one feature (see Charting Features).

This example shows a patient obviously dominant in red (sycosis)

YELLOW	RED	BLUE
Freckles	Hairline	Recessed eyelids
Front teeth	Smile	Dimples
	F/head	
	Bridge	
	Chin	
	Eyes	

Check all features and rate them to the appropriate primary miasm or leave un-rated if they fall within an average range. These ranges are discussed in the relevant facial feature sections.

THEMES

Another point to consider is the influence of the patient's story upon the practitioner. Themes go hand in hand with facial analysis and it was not long after the system developed that themes became obvious. Each miasmatic group has a unique outlook on life, and the events and circumstances they draw are equally distinct.

It is easy for themes to cloud objectivity. Once a practitioner has become 'convinced' of the miasm by the patient's story, they will 'see' facial features confirming that decision. If the practitioner has decided their patient is yellow, their eyes will see yellow facial features until 'forced' to reconsider.

In the past, I lost a lot of valuable time before realising I was working in the wrong miasm. You will know you are in the wrong group because your patient fails to respond. You have been careful in the selection process, you have taken a good case, and there are no missing links yet the patient fails to gain ground. Their continual failure to respond forces you to rethink the case. Another look at the patient's photographs – now through more objective eyes – reveals features that were previously overlooked or overstated. It now becomes obvious why your 'well chosen' yellow remedies failed – your patient is not yellow.

With every case that fails to respond

1. Recheck your photos and make sure the patient is in the right miasmatic group. If you are wrong, the whole case will be out. Every time your patient fails to respond this is the first thing to do. If your photos have been examined five or six times or they are unclear, then take another set

2. If you are confident of the miasm and confident of your case, recheck your previous repertorisations to see if one remedy keeps showing itself in the background.

3. If, on rechecking the miasm – provided you are happy with your case – you find your patient belongs to another miasmatic group, all that remains is to select the most appropriate remedy from the new miasmatic group. For example, there may be more red in your patient than previously noticed making them orange not yellow. Examining your previous repertorisations, (always keep a copy of every graph) you see Nux Vom. and Nat Mur. have always been near the top of every repertorisation. However, they were overlooked due to their miasmatic grouping. Read the materia medica on these two remedies carefully because one will do the job. With the miasm now accurately determined, orange remedies will succeed where yellow remedies failed.

CASE TAKING

Following nature's lead and applying facial analysis is a powerful adjunct in the clinic but even this means little if case taking is inadequate.

Some current thinking suggests we dig and delve to uncover the unconscious motivating force, but I disagree. Energy strong enough to influence and carve a pattern in life is energy that is easy to observe.

To understand the nature of personal energy we need to listen to a person's life story. Their energy will be seen in what they love to do, where they want to be, who they want to be with and what they make time for. Sometimes influencing energy may be an event rather than a focus. In this instance, it will be an event or series of events that are impacting or frequent. Take this information literally and at face value then find a rubric that best describes it.

For example, one recent patient had a life story which included the death of one of her parents while she was young and later on, the death of her husband in a car accident. She also works as a nurse in palliative care. In her case death must feature in the repertorisation. The question is, which rubric best describes this energy? Is it 'death -presentment of' or 'death -fear of '? – Because she has shown no signs of fear, 'death-presentment of ' was my choice.

Because there was so much death in her life when compared to the average person, what this woman thinks about death or her reaction to it is less consequential than the event itself. The well-known biblical statement 'seek and ye shall find' highlights the obvious nature of truth. Human beings love secrets and hidden truth, because secrets – especially those disguised as wisdom – elevate the status of the person who knows it. It is the typical school-yard – 'I know something you don't'. However, truth is never hidden, that's why all we have to do is 'seek' it. Truth is what exists, it is present and out there for all to see. Lies and secrets are what we keep hidden. Truth is transparent.

REPERTORISING

Repertorising like any other form of data input is reliant on the accuracy of the information fed into it. The repertory does not sift through information it simply arranges input. Accurate input means accurate output while incorrect input means incorrect output. Therefore, information to be repertorised must be accurate. If rubrics are so important – –what is a rubric?

A rubric is a physical symptom, modality, sensation, time, mental outlook or a state of being. Events and circumstances are also rubrics. Circumstance has often been overlooked as a rubric in repertorising even though it is often the strongest constant force, and this is a grave mistake.

The factors that determine whether a circumstance or symptom should become a rubric are

1. Frequency

2. Distinction

3. Impact

Frequency means regularity of occurrence, something that occurs more consistently than would otherwise be expected.

Distinction is like a mental PQRS, it is out of place, unexpected or unique.

Impact is an event or fear that is so influential it restructures how a patient lives their life. Something does not have to be a trend to be impacting.

Some examples of matching lifestyle to rubrics include:

Patient displays	Rubric to match
History of travelling	Desire to travel
History of abusive relationships	Violence
Feeling put down or humiliated	Ailments from mortification
History of 'bad luck' or accidents	Injuries, blows and bruises
Obsessive	Persistent thoughts
Argumentative	Quarrelsome
Laughing, making light of everything	Cheerful
Always working	Industrious

RESULTS

Like many modern day homoeopaths, I have a history of adaptation. Any system that offered help through the constitutional maze was worth a try. Unfortunately, many of these systems ended in me swapping one confusion for another. In the end I just stuck with standard 'classical' homoeopathy. Like most practitioners, I had my fair share of successes but, also like most practitioners, I had to spend more hours than I care to think about achieving each one.

I was a standard suburban homoeopath working extremely hard with my ego hanging by a thread. I did not want to give up homoeopathy yet at the same time I needed more from it. I needed more success and I needed willing patients. I needed a diary that had newly recommended patients combined with recent follow-ups, and patients happy to come back for their six monthly check-up. I needed to feel less guilty about charging money for patients who were not responding even though I was trying my best. Most of all I needed consistency. The boom and bust ride of patient success was wearing thin and I looked forward to the day when experience would grant me the things I needed. I knew it would all come when I finally had enough experience unfortunately; although I was gaining in experience, the consistency I craved never seemed to get any closer.

What I was looking for is what all homoeopaths are looking for – successful results. Our hope is that one day we will be able to put our knowledge into practice and finally be good at homoeopathy. Kent stated that it takes at least ten years to advance beyond the stage of novice and with standard 'classical' homoeopathy I think he is right. However, 'classical' homoeopathy does not include facial analysis and it is my firm belief that this system can cut ten years down to three. In three years, a practitioner using facial analysis will have results consistent with those normally gained by practitioners far more advanced. Early results are important to the profession otherwise there will be no one around to reach 'master' status as too many will leave because the out-put is too hard and the in-put too little. It is my sincere hope that facial analysis can help put a stop to this trend and that homoeopathy can once again proudly boast of its successes.

CHAPTER 23

Charting Features

Each feature showing a miasmatic influence is charted as either yellow (psora), red (sycosis) or blue (syphilis).

The purpose of charting facial features is to determine a patient's dominant miasm. As discussed in Appearance and Circumstance all have one dominant miasm and do so for life. During development when features change they change according to their dominant miasm. We have researched thousands of cases to determine at what point a miasm becomes dominant. The answer is two features more ahead of the next closest miasm. When one miasm is only one feature higher or lower than the next closest miasm it is regarded as equal in strength. In general a face will have between eight to twenty rated features.

The **dominant miasm** must be **2 points ahead** of the next miasm

- Where two miasms are within 1 point they are joined.
- Where three miasms are within 1 point of each other the lowest must still be 1 point away from the highest. If the lowest miasm is 2 points behind the highest drop it off the analysis.

Miasm = Yellow

The yellow features are 3 ahead of the closest primary miasm

YELLOW – 6	RED – 3	BLUE – 1
Freckles Front teeth prominent Ears – high Forehead – slopes back Chin – slopes back Smile – compact	Lips – full Hairline – straight Bridge – full	Teeth – overbite

Miasm = Red

The red features are 3 ahead of the closest primary miasm

YELLOW – 3	RED – 6	BLUE – 2
2 lines between eyes Forehead – slopes back Freckles	Gums show on smile Hairline – straight Bridge – straight Lips – full Teeth – even Ears stick out	Deep set eyes Asymmetry (eyes/chin)

Miasm = Blue

The blue features are 6 ahead of the closest primary miasm

YELLOW – 1	RED – 2	BLUE – 8
Ears – high	Nose – ball Chin – cleft	Eyes – upturned Eyes – recessed lids Chin – pointed Teeth – overbite Asymmetry (eyes/nose) Hairline – high Ears – large Bridge – indented

Miasm = Orange

The yellow and red features are ahead of the closest primary miasm. They are within 1 feature of each other therefore they are of equal strength. They are stronger than the blue miasm by 2 features so they dominate. The red and yellow miasms are of equal strength because they are separated by only one feature. The blue miasm is two features behind and therefore not influential enough to count.

YELLOW – 5	RED – 5	BLUE – 3
Eyes – small	Brow – full	Asymmetry (nose/chin)
Nose – bump	Hairline – straight	Eyes – recessed lids
Forehead – slopes back	Hairline – low	Cheek – dimple
Ears – low	Smile – full	
Mouth – small	Teeth – even	

Miasm = Green

The yellow and blue features are within 1 feature of each other therefore they are of equal strength. The red miasm is not strong enough to be of consideration.

YELLOW – 4	RED – 1	BLUE – 5
Mouth – small	Teeth – gaps	Asymmetry (ears/eyes)
Lines – under eyes		Asymmetry (mouth/chin)
Hairline – M shape		Forehead – dip inwards
Lips – thin		Hairline – high
		Teeth – crooked

Miasm = Purple

The red and blue features are ahead of the next closest primary miasm. Neither is stronger (by 2 features) than the other therefore they are of equal strength. The yellow miasm is not influential enough to consider.

YELLOW – 1	RED – 6	BLUE – 6
Nose – bump	Teeth – even	Asymmetry (ears/smile)
	Smile – full	Asymmetry (eyes/chin)
	Nose – wide	Teeth – inward
	Hairline – crowded	Cheeks – dimples
	Brow – full	Bridge – indented
	Forehead – straight	Ears – small

Miasm = Brown

The yellow, red and blue features are all within 1 feature of one another. Neither is stronger (by 2 features) than the other – they are of equal strength

YELLOW – 5	RED – 5	BLUE – 4
Nose – down-turned	Brow – full	Forehead – dips inward
Forehead – slopes back	Gums – show on	Eyes – deep set
Hairline – widows	smile	Eyes – recessed lids
peak	Teeth – even	Asymmetry (eyes/
Lines – below eyes	Smile – full	mouth)
Lines – 2 between eyes	Lips – full	

Examples Of Adding Up The Features

Miasm = Brown

The yellow, red and blue features are all within 1 feature of one another. Neither is stronger (by 2 features) therefore they are of equal strength

YELLOW	RED	BLUE
5	5	6

Miasm = Brown

The yellow, red and blue features are all within 1 feature of one another. Neither is stronger (by 2 features) than the other – they are of equal strength

YELLOW	RED	BLUE
3	4	3

Miasm = Brown

The yellow, red and blue features are all within 1 feature of one another. Neither is stronger (by 2 features) than the other – they are of equal strength

YELLOW	RED	BLUE
5	6	5

Miasm = Purple

The red and blue features are within 1 feature of one another. Neither is stronger (by 2 features) than the other therefore they are of equal strength but the blue miasm is stronger (by 2 or more features) than the yellow so the yellow doesn't count. This is an example of a "cusp" situation. If there is one more yellow feature the patient is brown.

YELLOW	RED	BLUE
3	4	5

Miasm = Purple

The red and blue features are within 1 feature of one another. Neither is stronger (by 2 features) than the other therefore they are of equal strength but the red miasm is stronger (by 2 or more features) than the yellow so the yellow doesn't count

YELLOW	RED	BLUE
3	6	5

Miasm = Green

The yellow and blue features are within 1 feature of one another.

Neither is stronger (by 2 features) than the other therefore they are of equal strength but the blue miasm is stronger (by 2 or more features) than the red so the red doesn't count. This is an example of a "cusp" situation. If there was one more red feature this patient would be brown. Examine the features very carefully

YELLOW	RED	BLUE
5	4	6

Miasm = Green

The yellow and blue features are within 1 feature or the same as one another. Neither is stronger (by 2 features) than the other therefore they are of equal strength and both are stronger (by 2 or more features) than the red so the red doesn't count

YELLOW	RED	BLUE
5	2	5

Miasm = Orange

The yellow and red features are within 1 feature or the same as one another. Neither is stronger (by 2 features) than the other therefore they are of equal strength and both are stronger (by 2 or more features) than the blue so the blue doesn't count

YELLOW	RED	BLUE
6	5	2

Miasm = Orange

The yellow and red features are within 1 feature or the same as one another. Neither is stronger (by 2 features) than the other therefore they are of equal strength and the red is stronger (by 2 or more features) than the blue so the blue doesn't count

YELLOW	RED	BLUE
4	5	3

Miasm = Blue

The blue features are stronger (by 2 features) than both the yellow and the red. However this is a double "cusp" situation where another yellow feature would equal green or another red feature would equal purple. Check the features carefully

YELLOW	RED	BLUE
3	3	5

Miasm = Blue

The blue features are stronger (by 2 features) than both the yellow and the red.

YELLOW	RED	BLUE
2	3	6

Miasm = Red

The red features are stronger (by 2 features) than both the yellow and the blue.

YELLOW	RED	BLUE
1	6	2

Miasm = Red

The red features are stronger (by 2 features) than both the yellow and the blue. This is an example of a "cusp" situation. If there was one more yellow feature this patient would be orange. Examine the features very carefully

YELLOW	RED	BLUE
3	5	2

Miasm = Yellow

The yellow features are stronger (by 2 features) than both the red and the blue.

YELLOW	RED	BLUE
7	4	2

Miasm = Yellow

The yellow features are stronger (by 2 features) than both the red and the blue. This is an example of a "cusp" situation. If there was one more blue feature this patient would be green. Examine the features very carefully

YELLOW	RED	BLUE
6		4

Facial analysis software - practitioner version is available to download from

http://www.soulandsurvival.org/wizard/download

Free 10 day trial - payment for continued use

CHAPTER 24

Taking Photos

The importance of using a digital camera cannot be underestimated. Features like asymmetry are more difficult to recognise with the naked eye and angles and size are easier to determine when using a camera. Investing in a camera is an investment in your clinical future. It is no different to investing in homoeopathic software and remedies.

WHICH CAMERA

For five years we have used a 2.2 megapixel camera but recently upgraded to a 7.2 megapixel camera and although the first camera was adequate it has to be said that our latest camera is better. In particular it allows for clearer zoom ups on teeth, hairlines and bridges.

WHAT TO TELL THE PATIENT

We have used this method on thousands of patients over the last few years. Some patients are amused but it is such an essential part of our practice that we wouldn't think of choosing a remedy until the patients' miasm (as assessed by facial analysis) has been determined. Photos are taken after the consultation has finished but as part of the introduction to the consultation the following is a recommended explanation.

"In this clinic we use facial analysis to determine your internal defense mechanism. After all of your symptoms have been described to me I will be taking some photos of your face and analyzing your facial structure through the computer. This information helps me to choose the best remedies for you"

After explaining the purpose of facial analysis most patients become involved and interested in the process.

TAKING THE PHOTOS

It is important that the patient is perfectly upright and straight. If the patient is not straight it is easy to misinterpret information or miss an emphasis or feature. With a digital camera you can check each photo as they are taken and repeat them again if required. It is easier if the patient sits in a chair especially if they are taller than you as this will allow you to be exactly horizontal to them with the camera. Remember if you take the photos either looking up or looking down at the patient all the angles will be false.

Many people naturally hold their head to one side or have a raised or lowered chin position. Ask the patient to sit up straight and keep asking them to move their head to the left or right or up or down until it is as level as possible. Then take the photo whilst asking them to hold that position. A tripod can be useful in keeping the camera level but is not essential.

FIVE* ESSENTIAL PHOTOS

Originally we only took three photos but as the system has developed we recognise the importance of taking five photos as described below. Sometimes we take as many as ten but this is only because we need to repeat one of the five until we are happy with that particular photo. Where possible take the photos against a plain light background as this makes them easier to analyse.

> *2010 – 7 photos – add one "frown" photo to highlight lines between the eyes and one "growl" photo to highlight both top and bottom row of teeth
>
> Video on how to take photos
>
> http://www.soulandsurvival.org/content/hfa-how-take-photos

Photo 1 – Face on relaxed

The patient is sitting face on and is level on both sides and the chin is level. The expression is relaxed – ask them to hold them lips naturally without smiling. The hair should be around the ears so the height of the ears can be determined both front on and side on.

Photo 2 – Hairline

Have the patient sit face on and level on both sides with their chin also level. This photo determines the shape of the hairline so the hair needs to be pulled back. Even a slight fringe or piece of hair draping down over the forehead can give a distorted image so ensure the hair is pulled back properly. Many men have their hair cut short or are balding so their hairline is easy to determine. Women and children often need to pull their hair back. Hairbands can be used although having the patient use both hands to pull back the hair seems to give the best image especially as they are pulling their hair more tightly so the hairline becomes clearly visible. Remind them to keep their head straight even though their arms are up.

Photo 3 – Smile and teeth

Ask the patient to drop their arms and have them smile as broadly as possible. Many patients do not smile very well when in front of the camera and need coaxing. If they are unable to smile have them grimace so that their teeth become visible. The compact smile (yellow) is often not seen in this photo and must be determined during the consultation. See the section on smiles for examples.

Photo 4 – Left profile

Whilst they are still seated have the patient swivel sideways in their chair at right angles to the camera. Again ensure that they are sitting up straight and that their chin is level. Their hair must be both pulled back from the forehead and pulled back from the ears. A hair-band is useful for this photo but they can use their arm to pull back their fringe. However their arm must be pulled back out of view of the profile or their profile will be more difficult to see in the final photo.

Once this position has been established ask them to slowly turn to their left. Watch the eye and the bridge of nose and when the furthest eye appears ask them to stop turning left. Now ask them to slowly turn back to their right whilst observing their furthest eye. Once this eye disappears from sight and the bridge is as close to 90 degrees to the camera as possible ask them to stop and hold still whilst the photo is taken. If the patient turns too far to their right during this process have them turn back to their left until they are 90 degrees to the camera*.

Photo 5 – Right profile

Whilst still seated have the patient swivel sideways in their chair in the opposite direction at right angles to the camera. Their hair must be both pulled back from the forehead and pulled back from the ears. Again ensure that they are sitting up straight and that their chin is level. A hair-band is useful for this photo but they can use their arm to pull back their fringe. However their arm must be pulled back out of view of the profile or their profile will be more difficult to see in the final photo.

Once this position has been established ask them to slowly turn to their right. Watch the eye and the bridge of nose and when the furthest eye appears ask them to stop turning right. Now ask them to slowly turn back to their left whilst observing their furthest eye. Once this eye disappears from sight and the bridge is as close to 90 degrees to the camera as possible ask them to stop and hold still whilst the photo is taken. If the patient turns too far to their left during this process have them turn back to their right until they are 90 degrees to the camera*.

SUMMARY

- Seat the patient
- Keep head level in all directions
- Pull hair back from forehead, ears and profile for photos 2, 4 & 5
- Request the broadest smile possible or an open mouth to show teeth
- Take the profile shots as close to 90 degrees as possible

*2010 – the profile position can be achieve through the patient sitting still and the camera operator moving side to side until they can see the bridge is at exactly 90 degrees – the more accurate the photos the easier and more accurate the analysis.

WHAT DOESN'T SHOW WELL IN PHOTOS

- **Facial lines** – due to the two dimensional nature of photos these lines are much easier to see when the patient is animated during the consultation. Make a note to include in your facial analysis. If you ask the patient to frown the lines between the eyes will become more apparent, however only include where they show strongly during this pose. Nearly everyone has some type of crease between the eyes when they frown but it must show strongly.

- **Skin markings** – freckles in particular may not show well but be quite apparent during the consultation.

- **Compact smile** – often more visible when the patient smiles naturally so will be seen during the consultation unless the patient smiles fully for the camera.

- **Cosmetic surgery** – remember to ask – the features **PRIOR** the surgery are the only ones worth analysing. A bump removed from a nose or teeth that used to be crooked are important pieces of information. Have the patient describe what their teeth or face used to be like - most will remember clearly. Old photos prior to the surgery can be helpful.

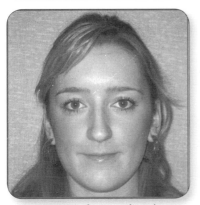

CORRECT – front on and straight

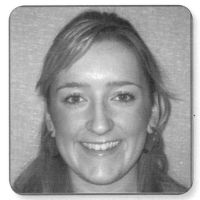

CORRECT – front on and smiling

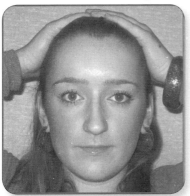

CORRECT – front on holding back hair

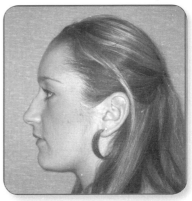

CORRECT – profile, left side of face*

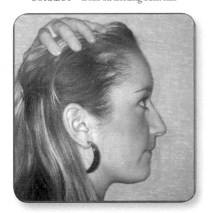

CORRECT – profile, right side of face with hair held back and arm held behind left side of head

*As this patient has her hair tied back it wasn't necessary for her to hold her hair back.

TAKING PHOTOS – COMMON MISTAKES

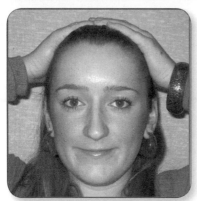

INCORRECT – head slightly turned

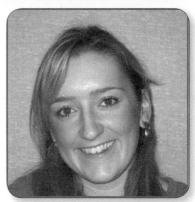

INCORRECT – head to one side

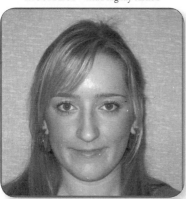

INCORRECT – chin is too low

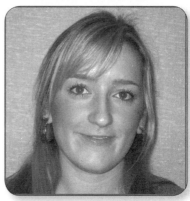

INCORRECT – head to one side

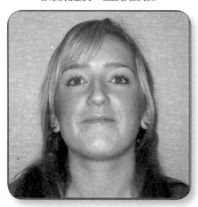

INCORRECT – chin too high

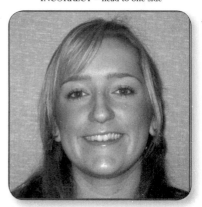

INCORRECT – head tilted up and back

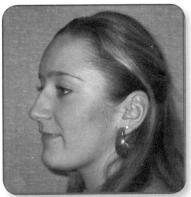

INCORRECT – head towards camera

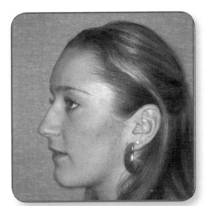

INCORRECT – head towards camera

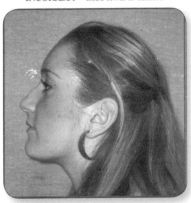

INCORRECT – chin too high

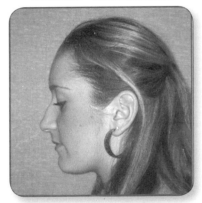

INCORRECT – chin too low

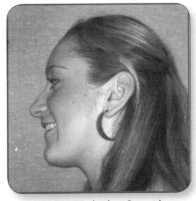

INCORRECT – head too far to right

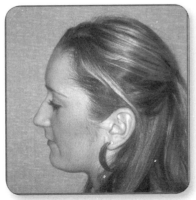

INCORRECT – head too far to left

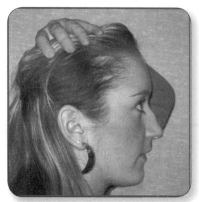

INCORRECT – elbow obstructing profile

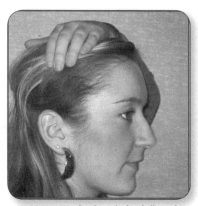

INCORRECT – head crooked and elbow obstructing profile

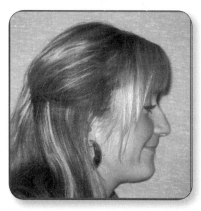

INCORRECT – hair covering ear and profile and chin too low

INCORRECT = taking a photo from too far away – remember to use the zoom or be close enough for face to be dominant in the screen

ABOUT THE PHOTOGRAPHS

Photographs as well as sketched illustrations feature throughout this book to show the feature in detail (sketch) as well as how it looks in real life (photo). Each photo chosen is a good 'real life' representation of the feature discussed however, it does not always come out looking that way in print. The reasons for this include

1. Photographs are flat – not three dimensional

2. To fit on the page, photos are shrunk to a much smaller size

3. Photographs are black and white and so miss natural skin tones

4. Definition is lost when printing a photo to standard paper

With all these factors in mind, do not be confused if you find the photographs a bit difficult to decipher at first. This difficulty is to be expected and is the reason behind the creation of this book. Appearance and Circumstance used photos as its instructional guide because at that time – being my first book – I was unaware of the difficulties of working with photos. With the expertise of hindsight Homoeopathic facial analysis' addresses this shortcoming by providing detailed illustrations as its main means of teaching.

It is still my belief that real life examples are beneficial and for this reason, photos are still included in this work.

CHAPTER 25

Children

Facial analysis is an important and useful tool for patients of any age. Children however pose their own special set of problems that need to be understood as part of the analysis.

Posing for photos

Most children under the age of four (and some quite a bit older) cannot sit still for long enough for a good set of photos to be taken. If the child will sit on a separate chair to have their photo taken the parent can help by holding the hair back and keeping the head firm. Babies and toddlers should be held on the parent's lap whilst you hold the camera freehand and move around until their image is centred. Often the child will follow your movements so the parent needs to help by distracting them with toys. Explain to the parent the five photos required so they can help to pose the child. It is common to use the information that has been gained by the naked eye more than the photos.

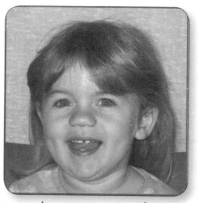

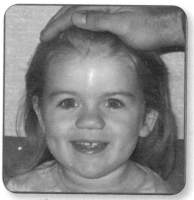

A common pose – not straight

The parent helps to straighten
the child and hold back the hair

CHANGING FEATURES

Many babies have an indented bridge of the nose to aid in feeding so do not use this feature under eighteen months unless it is very pronounced. As we grow from a baby to a young adult changes occur with our facial features. It is common for the nose and teeth to change shape over time. After seven years of analysing faces, we have observed that although these changes occur, another feature will also change resulting in the same miasm showing on the face. DNA influences features that are in turn influenced by the miasm. It remains the same miasm, no matter what changes occur.

NUMBER OF FEATURES

Both baby fat and the moving child make analysis more difficult than with adults. It is common for an analysis to contain as little as five to seven features in total. However if analysed correctly the result will be the same no matter how many features. It is prudent to consider that due to the lesser amount of features and the difficulties in analysing them, other close miasms should be considered.

TEETH

More than any other feature teeth will demonstrate many
changes. It is still interesting that the baby teeth will often display
the miasm in just the same way as the teeth of the older child.
Slight spaces (red), serrated edges (blue), more dominant front
teeth (yellow) will still be seen. The most difficult age is when
the teeth are falling out, usually around five to seven. Then of
course single gaps will be seen but these should not be rated.

HAIRLINES

Widow's Peak — Yellow

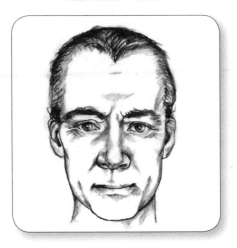

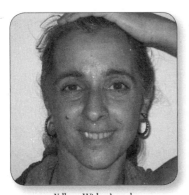

Yellow -Widow's peak

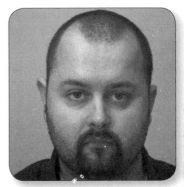

Yellow - M shape

The widow's peak is where the fringe of the hairline creates a downward triangular peak. This peak may come to a sharp point or be rounded to form an M.

HAIRLINES

Widow's Peak — Yellow

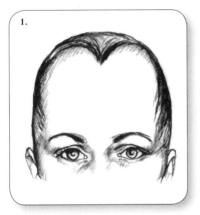

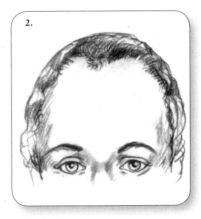

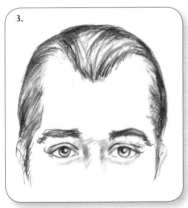

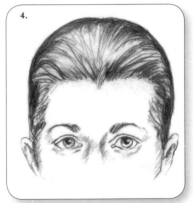

1. A triangular peak (yellow). This hairline will get two points. Widows peak (yellow) and high hairline (blue)

2. A cowlick either centred or off to one side (yellow). This hairline will get two points. Widows peak (yellow) and high hairline (blue)

3. An M shaped hairline seen mostly in men where the hair on the temple has receded back (yellow). This hairline will get two points. Widows peak (yellow) and high hairline (blue)

4. A small widow's peak in an otherwise straight hairline. This hairline will get two points. Widow's peak (yellow), straight hairline (red)

HAIRLINES

Straight - Red

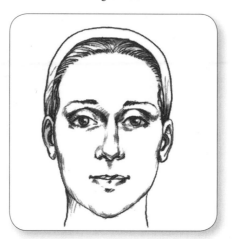

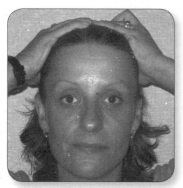

Red- Hairline straight

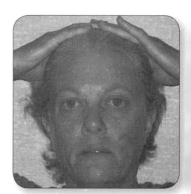

Red- Hairline straight (oval)

Many features in red are straight including the hairline. Provided the overall impression is of a straight line each hair does not have to be perfectly even.

HAIRLINES

Straight — Red

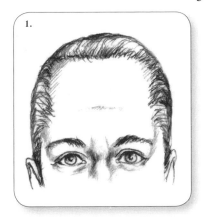

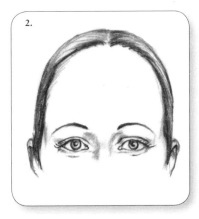

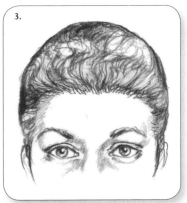

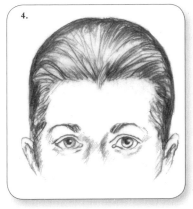

1. A straight horizontal hairline across the forehead that is also high. This hairline will get two points. Straight (red) and high (blue)

2. A straight and high hairline giving an oval shape. This hairline will get two points. Straight (red) and high (blue)

3. A straight hairline that is also low. This hairline will get two points. Straight (red) and low (red)

4. A straight hairline with a widow's peak. This hairline will get two points. Straight (red) and widow's peak (yellow). The height is average

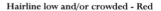

HAIRLINES

Hairline low and/or crowded - Red

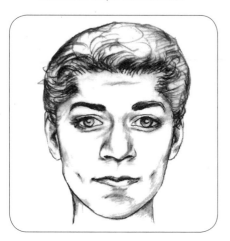

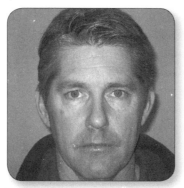

Red - Hairline crowded

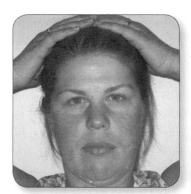

Red - Hairline low

Crowded - a crowded hairline is the term given to describe a hairline that encroaches inward on both sides of the forehead and temples. In this feature, the hairline of the temples extends inward past the outer end of each eyebrow.

Low - a low hairline is approximately ½ cm below the main curve of the forehead. An average hairline ranges from level with this curve to ½ cm above it.

HAIRLINES

Hairline low and/or crowded — Red

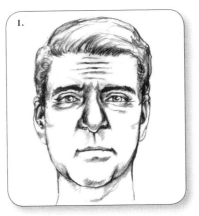

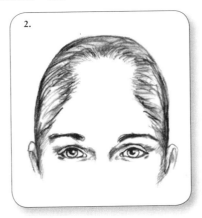

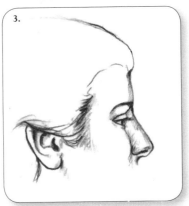

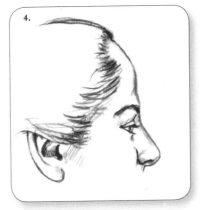

1. A low and straight hairline. This hairline will get two points. Low (red) and straight (red).

2. A crowded and higher hairline that gives the forehead a narrow appearance. This hairline will get two points. Crowded (red) and high (blue).

3. A low hairline on profile (red).

4. A crowded hairline on profile (red). This hairline will get two points. Crowded (red) and high (blue).

HAIRLINES

Hairline high - Blue

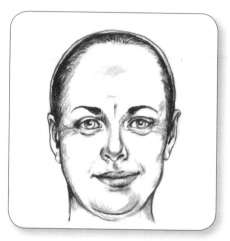

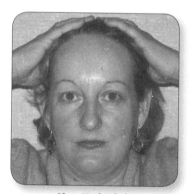

Blue - Hairline high

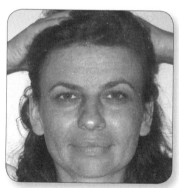

Control- Height not rated

A high hairline means the edge is set back past the natural curve of the scalp. This lengthens the distance between the eyebrows and the hairline often making the forehead seem longer. A hairline is high regardless of shape.

HAIRLINES

Hairline high — Blue

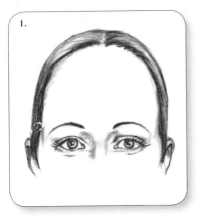
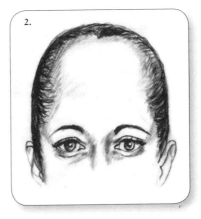
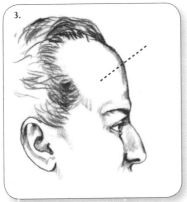
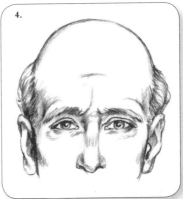

1. A high but straight hairline giving an overall oval impression. This hairline will get two points. High (blue) and straight (red)

2. A high hairline with a widow's peak. This hairline will get two points. High (blue) and widow's peak (yellow)

3. A high hairline showing the start of the hairline above the curve of the scalp, as seen on profile (blue)

4. Baldness (blue)

FOREHEADS

Forehead sloped - Yellow

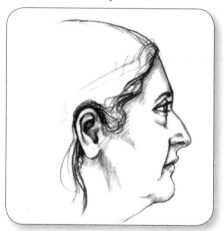

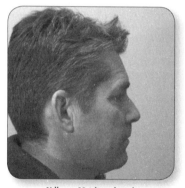

Yellow - Hairline sloped

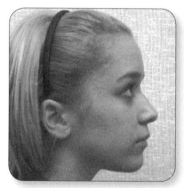

Control- curved not sloped

The measuring point for the forehead is from between the eyebrows. From this starting point the angle and shape of the forehead is assessed. If a forehead is yellow, it will slope backwards in a straight line at an angle of 12 or greater. If the forehead curves backwards it is blue. If the forehead is 11 or less it is red*.

*Footnote 2010 – if the head is tilted even slightly – up or down from its natural level the angle of the forehead will change. Whenever a forehead is between 10 and 12 degrees it could be red or yellow – put a question mark and factor into the total analysis

FOREHEADS

Forehead sloped — Yellow

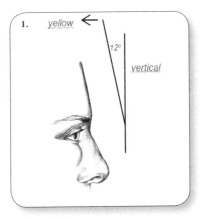
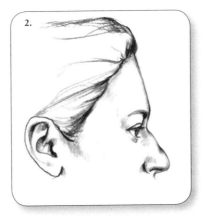

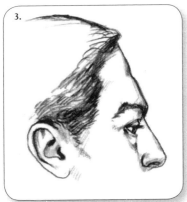
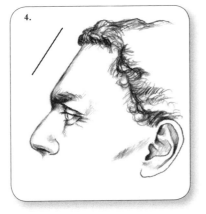

1. The reference line that divides yellow from red – 12 or greater is yellow.

2. The most commonly seen example of the yellow forehead.

3. A sloped and indented forehead. This forehead will get two points. Sloped (yellow) and indented (blue).

4. A sloped forehead at an acute angle (yellow).

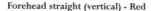

FOREHEADS

Forehead straight (vertical) - Red

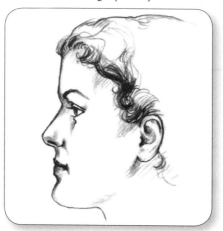

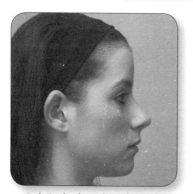

Red- Forehead straight (and vertical)

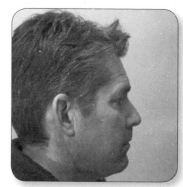

Control-straight (and sloped)

Using between the eyes as the starting place, the red forehead is a straight or almost vertical line (between 0 and 11) from this point. A forehead must curve at some point to form the top of the head. The last 20% of the forehead is often curved but as long as the first 80% is straight this type of forehead is red.

FOREHEADS

Forehead straight (vertical) — Red

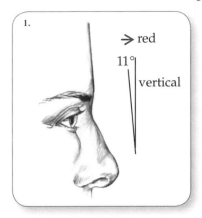

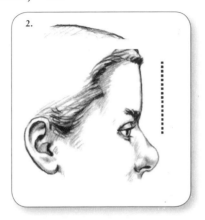

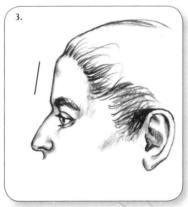

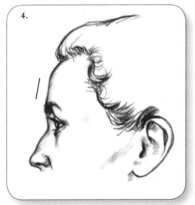

1. The reference line that divides red from yellow – from vertical to 11° is red.

2. The most commonly seen example of the red forehead.

3. The last 20% of the forehead is curved but as 80% of the forehead is straight it is still red.

4. The last 30 – 40 % of this forehead is curved so this forehead will get two points. Straight (red) and curved (blue). Note this angle is 10° (red).

FOREHEADS

Forehead curved - Blue

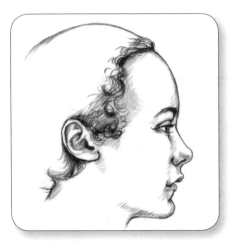

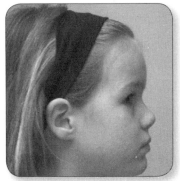

Blue - Forehead curved

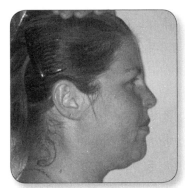

Control- not curved

The curved forehead of blue is a continuous arc extending from between the eyes to the hairline. The curves found in the blue forehead range from a gentle continuous arc, to a semi-circle. When it reaches this degree, the forehead takes on a bulging appearance.

FOREHEADS

Forehead curved — Blue

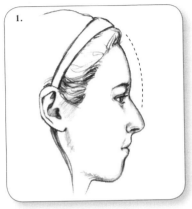

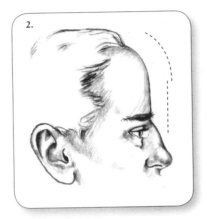

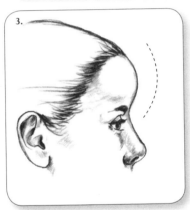

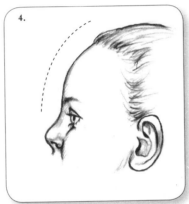

1. A gentle backward curve, because of its curved shape this forehead is blue.

2. A forehead that is both curved and straight. Straight (vertical) for the first 60% then curved for the last 40%. This forehead will get two points. Curved (blue) and straight (red).

3. An outward bulging curve (blue).

4. A curved forehead seen in a child (blue). Even though this forehead slopes back, it is still blue, because it is curved.

FOREHEADS

Forehead indented - Blue

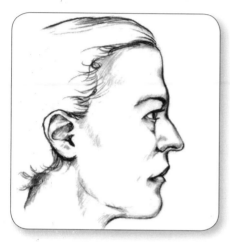

This forehead takes closer examination than many facial features, because it resembles the sloping forehead of yellow. However, instead of one straight continuous line, the indented blue forehead is actually wavy not straight therefore, it is two small joined curves rather than one long arc.

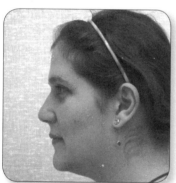

Blue - Forehead indented

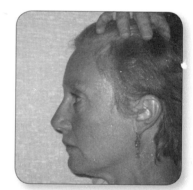

Blue - Forehead curved

Using between the eyes as the starting point, notice the forehead dips in approximately one third the way up toward the hairline. It then curves outward at a slight angle to join the top of the head. The difference between an indented forehead and a brow

- The indented forehead looks like a continuous wave.
- A brow is a semi-circular bony projection along or just above the eyebrows.

FOREHEADS

Forehead indented — Blue

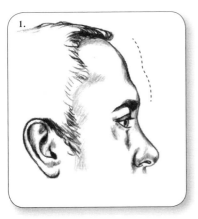

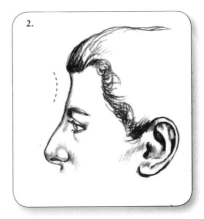

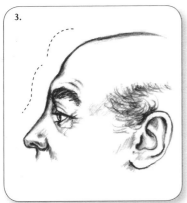

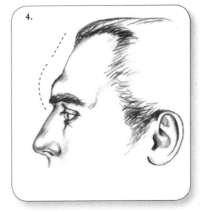

1. Indented forehead curving backwards (blue).

2. Indented forehead with a concave curve (blue).

3. Two curves with an indentation (blue). Compare with picture 4

4. NOT BLUE – Semi-circular brow joining a straight sloped forehead. This can look very similar to the example in number 3. This forehead will get two points. Brow (red) and straight sloped (yellow). A forehead that has both a brow (red) and a curve above the brow (blue) also exists.

FOREHEADS

Forehead brow - Red

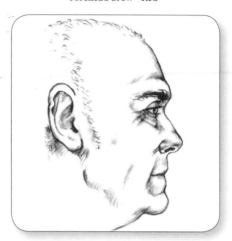

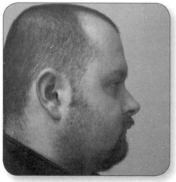

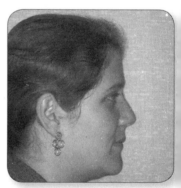

Red - Forehead brow   Control - Indented - no brow

A brow is a bony projection that begins level to the eyebrows and gently curves outward extending upward into the forehead for approximately one to two centimetres to join with the forehead. It is separate from the forehead. The red brow differs from the indented forehead of blue because it is a semicircular outward curve rather than a concave indentation.

FOREHEADS

Forehead brow — Red

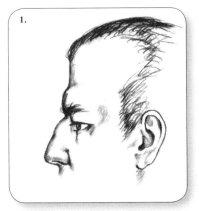

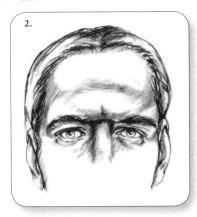

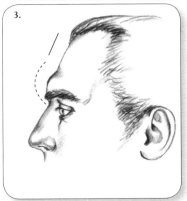

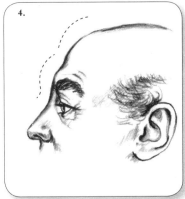

1. A brow with a straight vertical forehead. This forehead will get two points. Brow (red) and straight vertical (red).

2. A brow from a frontal view. From this position the forehead appears indented but on profile it is the brow that is strong (red) not the forehead.

3. A brow with a straight sloped (yellow) forehead. This forehead will get two points. Brow (red) and straight sloped (yellow). Compare with picture 4.

4. NOT RED – two curves with an indentation. This can look very similar to the example in number 3. This forehead is blue only, it does not have the outward curve that defines a brow.

BRIDGE OF NOSE

Bridge full- Red

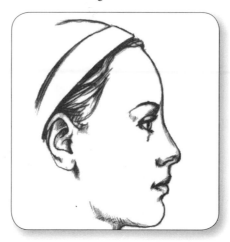

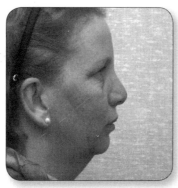

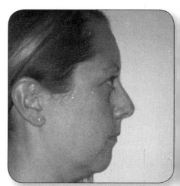

Red- Bridge full   Control - bridge not rated

The term bridge in this context is the point between the forehead and the commencement of the nose. There are two ways of viewing this fullness.

1. In a full or vertical bridge, the bone of the nose begins between the eyebrows. It does not have an inward curve
2. Full bridge is also used to describe the distance between the eye and the bone of the nose on profile

BRIDGE OF NOSE

Bridge full — Red

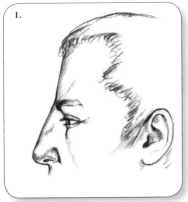

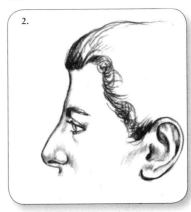

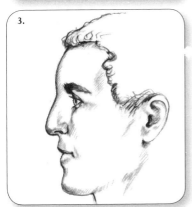

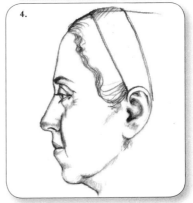

1. The bridge in this example extends directly downward from a position slightly higher than the middle of the eyebrows. This gives the impression that the nose starts from the forehead (red).

2. The bridge extends from the more standard middle of the eyebrow position before extending outward into the nose (red).

3. Although there is a curve in the bridge, the distance between the eye and the bridge of the nose is greater than average (red). See picture 4.

4. AVERAGE BRIDGE – not rated. Both the full and indented bridge are measured against this point. Anything more full or straight is red and anything less is indented (blue).

BRIDGE OF NOSE

Bridge indented - Blue

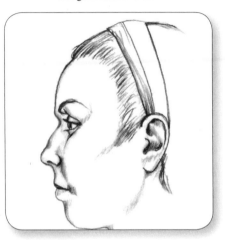

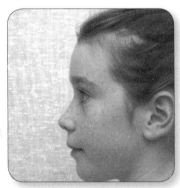

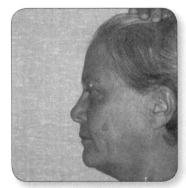

Blue - Bridge indented   Control- Bridge not rated

The term bridge in this context is the point between the forehead and the commencement of the nose. With an indented bridge the nose curves or cuts inward toward the eyes before extending outward to the nose. The bridge on profile has a definite concave appearance.

BRIDGE OF NOSE

Bridge indented — Blue

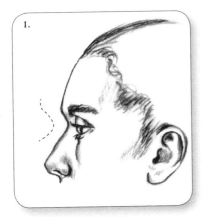

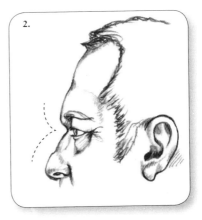

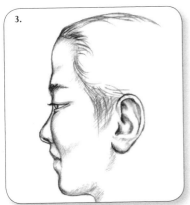

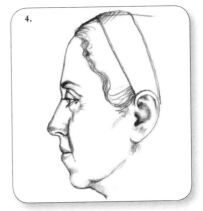

1. A gentle continuous inward curve (blue).

2. A smaller but sharper 'cut' creating a sideways V appearance between the forehead and the nose (blue).

3. No bridge at all, where the bone of the nose is almost nonexistent like that of many new born babies (blue).

4. AVERAGE BRIDGE – not rated. Both the full and indented bridge are measured against this point. Anything more full or straight is red and anything less is indented (blue).

EYES

Eyes down-turned - Yellow

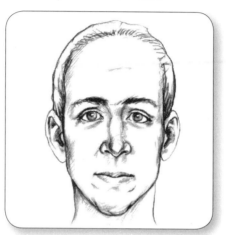

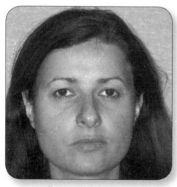

Yellow- Eyes down-turned

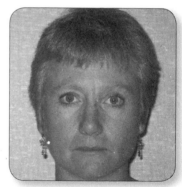

Control- eye shape not rated

Down-turned eyes slope downward at a more pronounced angle than the first half of the upper eyelid. Down-turned eyes occur regardless of whether the eyelids are full or recessed.

EYES

Eyes down-turned — Yellow

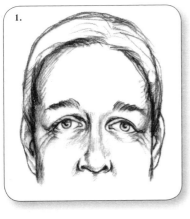

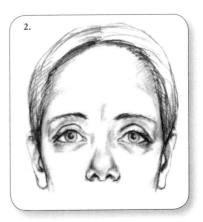

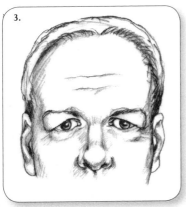

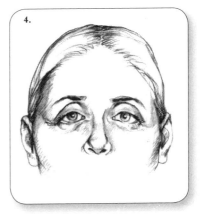

1. A commonly seen example of down-turned eyes (yellow).

2. A subtle example, but still regarded as down-turned (yellow).

3. Down-turned eyes with recessed lids. These eyes will get two points. Down-turned (yellow) and recessed lids (blue).

4. Down-turned eyes with full lids. These eyes will get two points. Down-turned eyes (yellow) and full lids (yellow).

EYES

Eyes close-set - Yellow

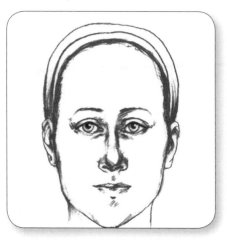

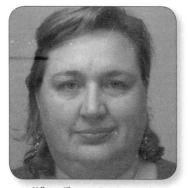

Yellow- Close-set (starting point)

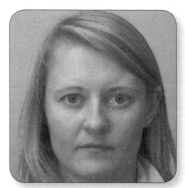

Control - not close-set

Close-set eyes are when the inner canthus of each eye appear closer to the bridge of the nose than average. No mathematical definition for close-set eyes exists so it relies on visual interpretation. It depends on a number of factors including the width of the face, the width of the nose, the length of the nose and the size of the eyes.

EYES

Eyes close-set — Yellow

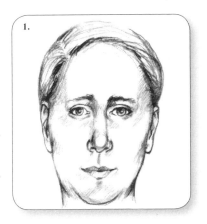

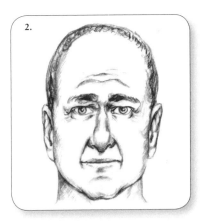

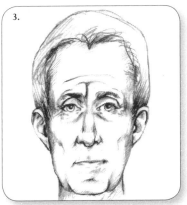

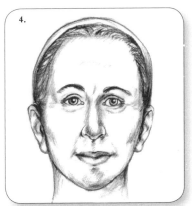

1. Close-set eyes (yellow).

2. Close-set eyes with recessed lids. These eyes will get two points. Close-set eyes (yellow) and recessed lids (blue).

3. Close set eyes with full lids. These eyes will get two points. Close-set (yellow) and full lids (yellow).

4. Close-set eyes which are small. These eyes will get two points. Close-set (yellow) and small eyes (yellow).

EYES

Eyes small - Yellow

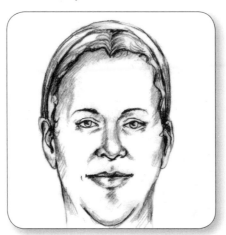

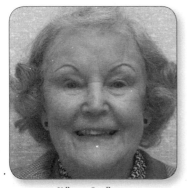

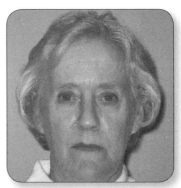

Yellow – Small eyes   Control – Size not rated

Small eyes are a visual interpretation in context with other facial features. There are no mathematical measurements. Eyes can appear small regardless of eye shape.

EYES

Eyes small - Yellow

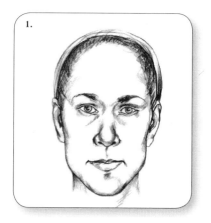

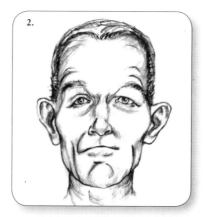

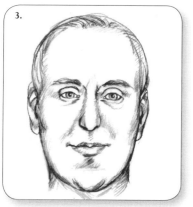

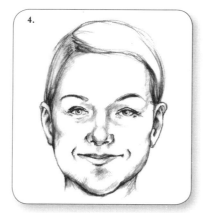

1. Small eyes that are also upturned. These eyes will get two points. Small eyes (yellow) and upturned eyes (blue)

2. Small eyes which are also down-turned. These eyes will get two points. Small eyes (yellow) and down-turned eyes (yellow)

3. Small eyes with full lids. These eyes will get two points. Small eyes (yellow) and full lids (yellow)

4. Small eyes (yellow)

EYES

Eyes full-lids - Yellow

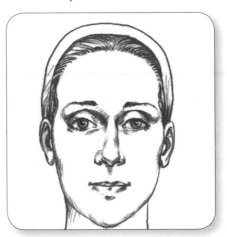

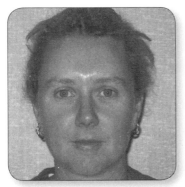

Yellow - Full lids (starting point)

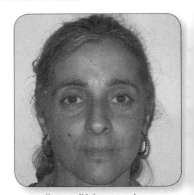

Yellow - Full lids commonly seen

Full lids extend over the eyeball covering an area of thirty percent or more. Picture one is where full lids begin. Anything less than this would not rate.

EYES

Eyes full-lids — Yellow

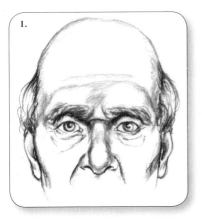 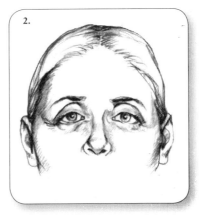

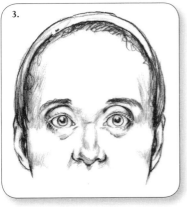 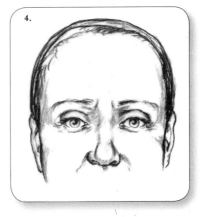

1. Full lids with deep-set eyes. These eyes will get two points. Full lids (yellow) and deep-set eyes (blue).

2. Full lids with down-turned eyes. These eyes will get two points. Full lids (yellow) and down-turned eyes (yellow).

3. Full lids with exophthalmic eyes. These eyes will get two points. Full lids (yellow) and exophthalmic eyes (red).

4. Full lids (yellow).

EYES

Eyes large - Red

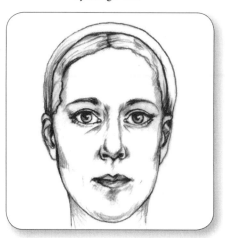

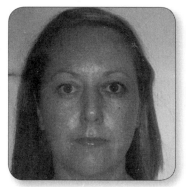

Red - Large eyes

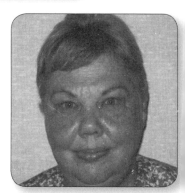

Control- Size not rated

Large eyes are a visual interpretation in context with other facial features. There are no mathematical measurements. Eyes can appear large regardless of eye shape.

EYES

Eyes large — Red

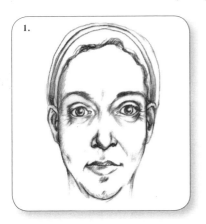

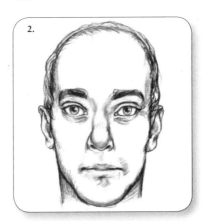

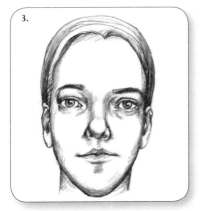

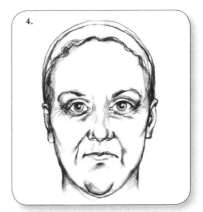

1. Large eyes which are also exophthalmic. These eyes will get two points. Large eyes (red) and exophthalmic eyes (red)

2. Large eyes that are also upturned. These eyes will get two points. Large eyes (red) and upturned eyes (blue)

3. Large eyes which are also wide-set. These eyes will get two points. Large eyes (red) and wide-set (blue)

4. Large eyes (red)

EYES
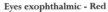

Eyes exophthalmic - Red

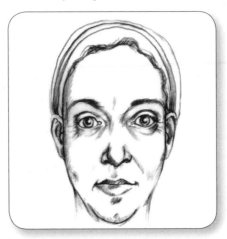

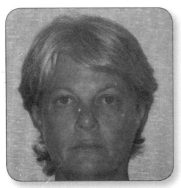

Red - Exophthalmic eyes

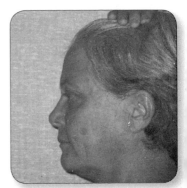

Red - Exophthalmic eyes on profile

There are two aspects to the exophthalmic eye.

- When the whole socket of the eye protrudes beyond the line of the face
- On profile the eyeball has a marked convex curve

Looking front on, exophthalmic eyes are noticed with the naked eye due to their three dimensional character. With a camera, they are best observed on profile. Exophthalmic eyes often give a 'staring' impression.

EYES

Eyes exophthalmic — Red

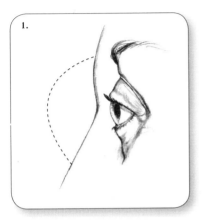

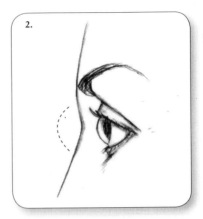

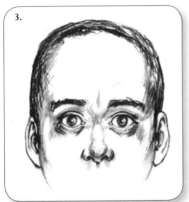

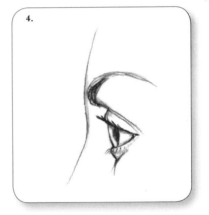

1. Exophthalmic eyes showing a protrusion of both the socket and the eyeball (red)

2. Convex curvature of the eye on profile (red) with a normal socket

3. Exophthalmic eyes frontal view (red)

4. Average curvature of the eye on profile – no rating

EYES

Eyes upturned- Blue

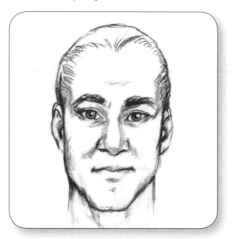

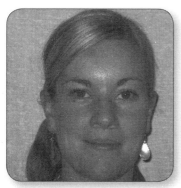
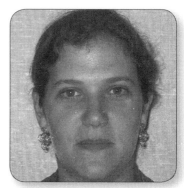

Blue - Upturned eyes   Control - Shape not rated

If a horizontal line is drawn from the inner canthus to the outer canthus, the level should be approximately even. When the outer canthus
is considerably higher, it gives the eye an 'upturned' appearance as
though the eye is slanting upwards at an angle.

EYES

Eyes upturned — Blue

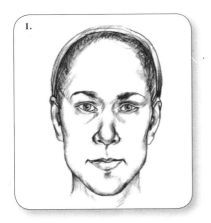

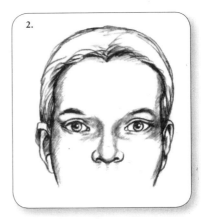

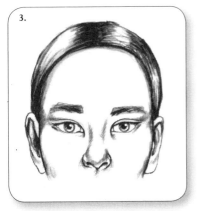

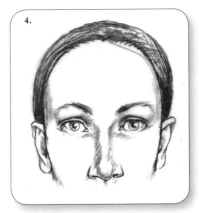

1. Upturned eyes that are also small. These eyes will get two points. Upturned eyes (blue) and small eyes (yellow)

2. Upturned eyes that are also wide-set. These eyes will get two points. Upturned eyes (blue) and wide-set eyes (blue)

3. Upturned eyes.

4. Upturned eyes (blue)

EYES

Eyes wide-set - Blue

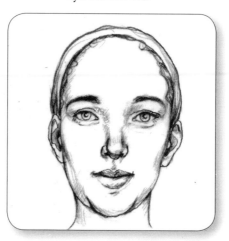

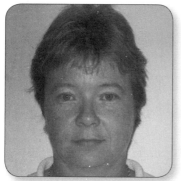

Blue - Wide-set eyes

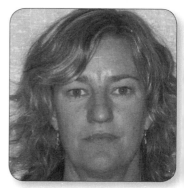

Control -Width not rated

Wide-set eyes are when the inner canthus of each eye appear further away from the bridge of the nose than average. No mathematical definition for wide-set eyes exists so it relies on visual interpretation. It depends on a number of factors including the width of the face, the width of the nose, the length of the nose and the size of the eyes. Wide-set eyes are often more observable 'face to face' than they are by photograph.

EYES

Eyes wide-set — Blue

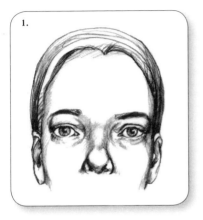

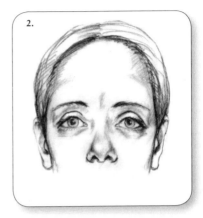

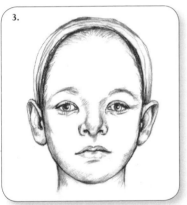

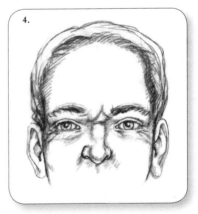

1. Wide-set eyes which are also large. These eyes will get two points. Wide-set eyes (blue) and large eyes (red)

2. Wide-set eyes which are also down-turned. These eyes will get two points. Wide-set eyes (blue) and down-turned eyes (yellow)

3. Wide-set eyes which are also small. This will get two points. Wide-set (blue) and small (yellow)

4. Wide-set eyes (blue)

EYES

Eyelids recessed- Blue

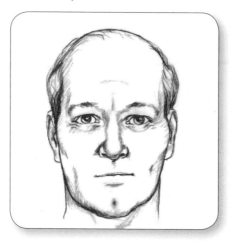

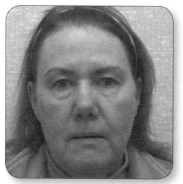

Blue -Eyelids recessed

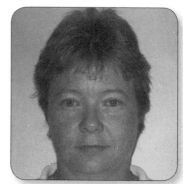

Control - Lids not rated

Many eyes have a layer or fold of skin referred to as the eyelid. If this fold or lid is not visible, it is recessed regardless of the shape of the eye. Usually the eyelashes are still visible. Recessed lids feature prominently amongst some races. Regardless of race or colour facial features are rated as they appear.

EYES

Eyelids recessed — Blue

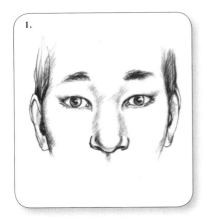

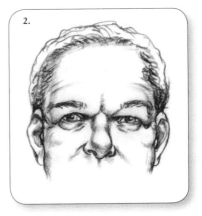

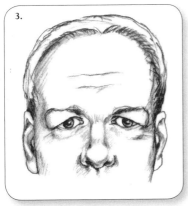

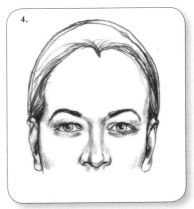

1. Recessed lids with upturned eyes. These eyes will get two points. Recessed lids (blue) and upturned eyes (blue)

2. Recessed lids with deep-set eyes. These eyes will get two points. Recessed lids (blue) and downturned eyes (yellow)

3. Recessed lids with down-turned eyes. These eyes will get two points. Recessed lids (blue) and down-turned eyes (yellow)

4. Recessed lids (blue)

EYES

Eyes deep-set - Blue

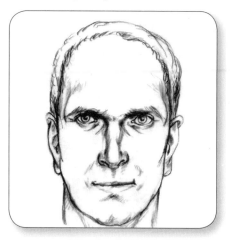

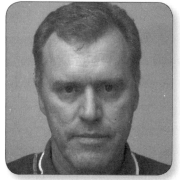

Blue - Deep-set eyes

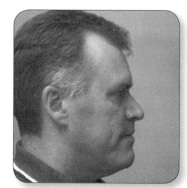

Blue- Deep-set eyes on profile

Deep-set eyes are a three dimensional facial feature and therefore not identified via a photograph easily. They are seen during the consultation. Deep-set eyes are different to recessed lids although both are blue features. Deep-set eyes are set further back into the skull rather than level with the face. Although sometimes seen with a heavy brow deep-set eyes are a separate feature to the brow.

EYES

Eyes deep-set — Blue

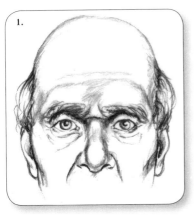

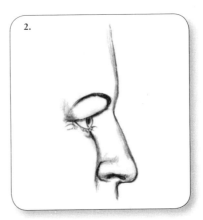

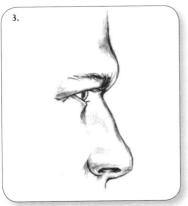

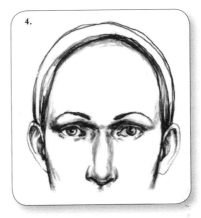

1. Deep-set eyes with full lids. These eyes will get two points. Deep-set eyes (blue) and full lids (yellow)

2. Deep-set eyes on profile (blue)

3. Deep-set eyes with a full brow on profile. These eyes will get two points. Deep-set eyes (blue) and full brow (red)

4. Deep-set eyes (blue)

NOSE

Nose bump - Yellow

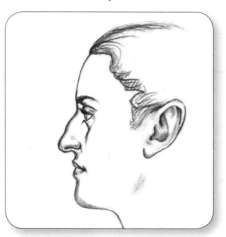

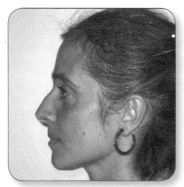

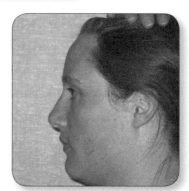

Yellow - Bump on nose   Control- Nose not rated

The bump of the nose is generally located in the upper third of the length of the nose on profile. However, in some cases it will be in the lower third. The bump itself will range from eye catching to just visible; however, whether blatant or subtle if the bump can be seen, it must be rated. A bump further down the nose, will give the nose an overall curved or 'hawkish' appearance.

NOSE

Nose bump — Yellow

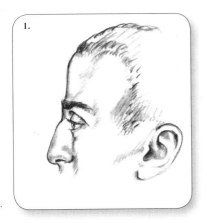

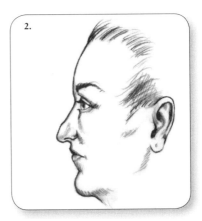

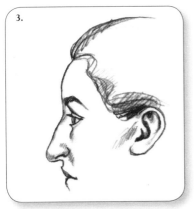

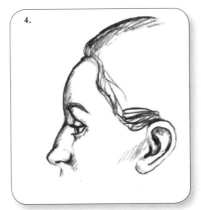

1. Bump on the nose - upper third (yellow).

2. Bump on the nose – lower third (yellow).

3. Bump on the nose and down-turned. This nose will get two points. Bump (yellow) and down-turned (yellow).

4. Bump on the nose – broad (yellow).

NOSE

Nose long downward/curved- Yellow

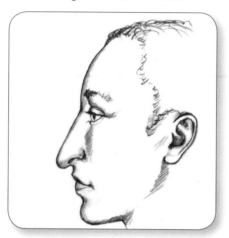

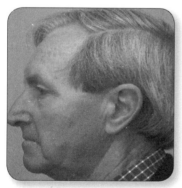

Yellow - Down-turned

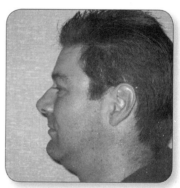

Control - Straight nose

There are two primary examples of the down-turned nose. The first is generally a longer nose where the tip of the nose is lower than the junction of the nose to the face; the second has a definite downward curve that is colloquially termed a 'hooked' nose.

NOSE

Nose long downward/curved — Yellow

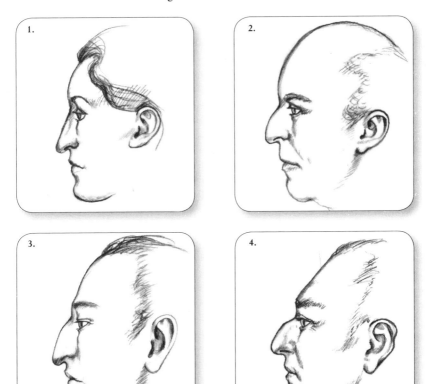

1. Down–turned nose (yellow).

2. Curved nose (yellow).

3. Down-turned with a bump. This nose will get two points. Down-turned (yellow) and bump (yellow).

4. Curved with a bump. This nose will get two points. Curved (yellow) and bump (yellow).

NOSE

Nose wide- Red

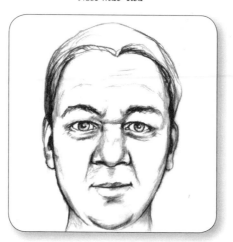

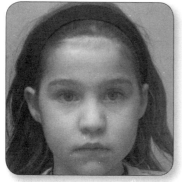

Red -Wide nose

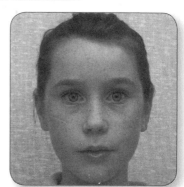

Control- Not wide

In a wide nose there are two types. The width of the nose has a broad surface area or the bone of the nose is average or thin while the end of the nose is wide.

NOSE

Nose wide — Red

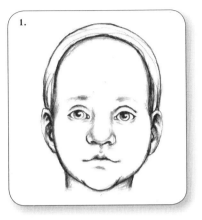

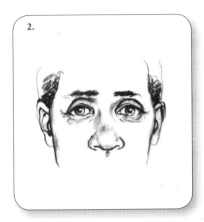

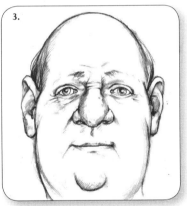

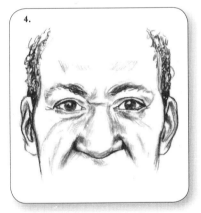

1. Broad nose down the whole length (red).

2. Thin bone of the nose with a wide base (red).

3. Bulbous or 'whiskey' nose (red).

4. Wide square base of the nose (red).

NOSE

Nose ball-shaped- Red

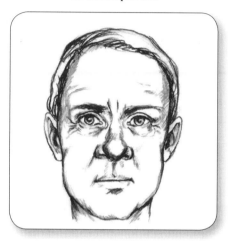

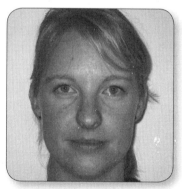

Red - Nose ball

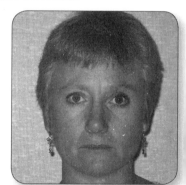

Control -Shape not rated

A ball shaped nose takes three main forms.

- The bone of the nose is straight while the end is rounded.
- The bridge is indented on profile with a round end.
- The nose has a standard shape with a round tip.

Sometimes the tip of the nose has an indentation or cleft, this is also red.

NOSE

Nose ball-shaped — Red

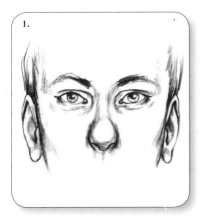

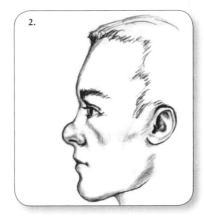

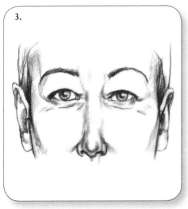

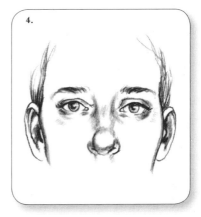

1. Ball nose with rounded end (red).

2. Ball nose with an indented bridge on profile. This nose will get two points. Ball (red) and indented bridge (blue).

3. The rounded tip at the end of an otherwise normal nose (red).

4. Ball sits forward of the nostrils (red).

CHEEKS

Prominent cheekbones and sunken cheeks - Blue

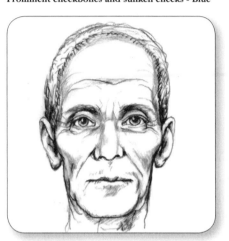

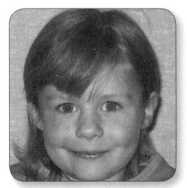

Blue- Prominent cheekbones

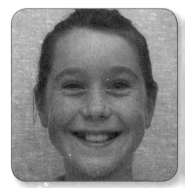

Control- No cheekbones visible

Cheekbones are high-lighted most while smiling; however, even when not smiling the cheekbones of some people can be quite defined. The cheekbones either create a U shape in the face or protrude out from the face as round balls in the cheeks. The key is the word 'prominence'. They must be distinctive.

CHEEKS

Prominent cheekbones and sunken cheeks — Blue

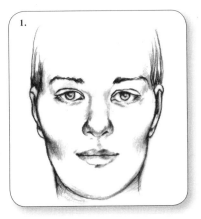

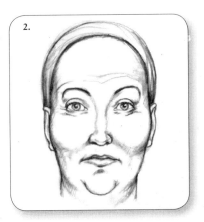

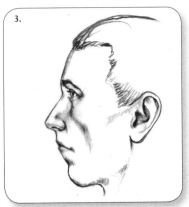

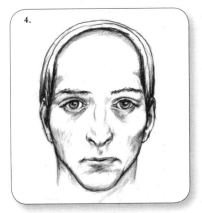

1. Prominent cheekbones (blue)

2. Prominent cheekbones with a 'fleshy' look (blue)

3. Sunken cheeks with a gaunt appearance (blue)

4. Sunken cheeks with prominent cheekbones. This will get two points. Prominent cheekbones (blue) and sunken cheeks (blue) – subtle example

MOUTH

Mouth small - Yellow

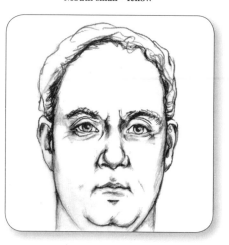

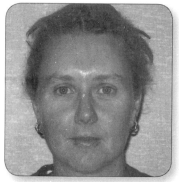

Yellow – Small mouth

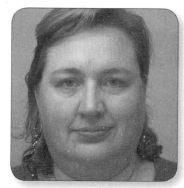

Control – Size not rated

If hypothetical lines are drawn downward in a straight line from the wings of the nose to the mouth, the 'average sized' mouth extends just beyond these lines. A small mouth lies inside these lines. The exception to this rule is when the base of the nose is wide in which case the mouth may be within normal limits but still fit into this criteria. However, by far the best indicator for a small mouth is when your eyes are drawn to it naturally.

MOUTH

Mouth small - Yellow

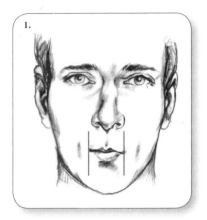

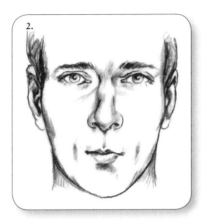

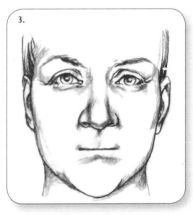

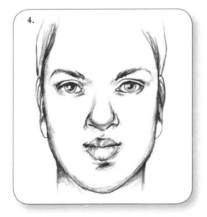

1. Small mouth showing the hypothetical lines (yellow).

2. Small mouth with normal lips (yellow).

3. Small mouth with thin lips. This mouth will get two points. Small mouth (yellow) and thin lips (yellow).

4. Small mouth with full lips. This mouth will get two points. Small mouth (yellow) and full lips (red).

MOUTH

Mouth wide - Red

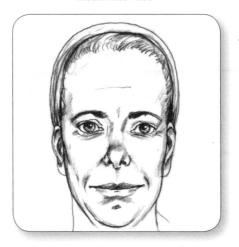

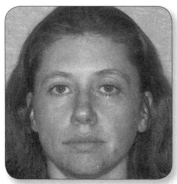

Red – Wide mouth

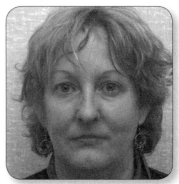

Control – Width of mouth not rated

If hypothetical lines are drawn downward in a straight line from the wings of the nose to the mouth, the 'average sized' mouth extends just beyond these lines. A wide mouth lies beyond these lines. The best indicator for a wide mouth is when your eyes are drawn to it naturally.

MOUTH

Mouth wide - Red

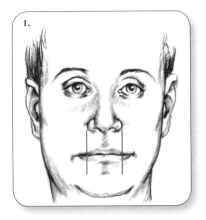

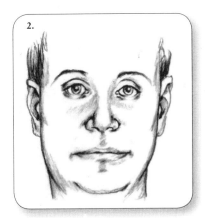

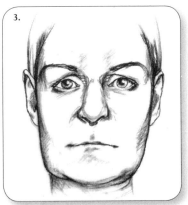

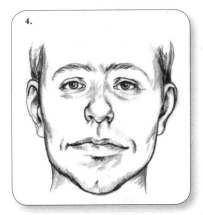

1. Wide mouth showing the hypothetical lines (red).

2. Wide mouth with normal lips (red).

3. Wide mouth with thin lips. This mouth will get two points. Wide mouth (red) and thin lips (yellow).

4. Wide mouth with full lips. This mouth will get two points. Wide mouth (red) and full lips (red).

LIPS

Lips thin - Yellow

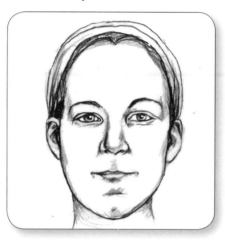

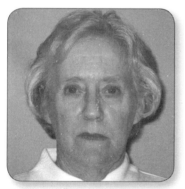

Yellow – Lips Thin

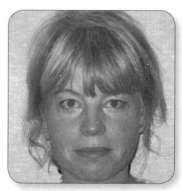

Control – Lips not rated

There are no limits or calculations to define thin lips. Thin lips, like many facial features are a visual impression. Lipstick can be a problem if it goes beyond the natural line of the lips so check the photo carefully. Assess the lips from a non-smiling photograph as smiling pulls the lips making them look thin.

LIPS

Lips thin - Yellow

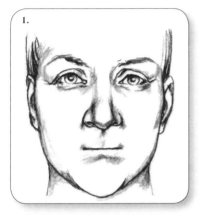
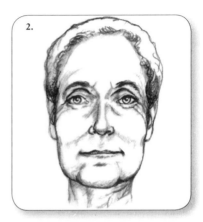

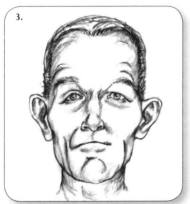
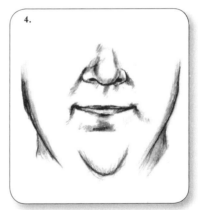

1. Thin lips with a small mouth. This mouth will get two points. Thin lips (yellow) and small mouth (yellow).

2. Thin lips with a wide mouth. This mouth will get two points. Thin lips (yellow) and wide mouth (red).

3. Thin lips with a down-turned mouth. This mouth will get two points. Thin lips (yellow) and down-turned mouth (blue).

4. Thin lips (yellow).

LIPS

Lips full - Red

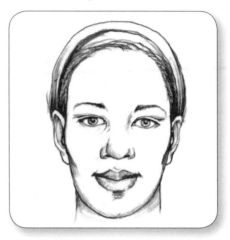

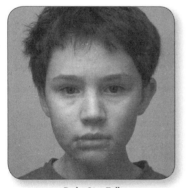

Red – Lips Full

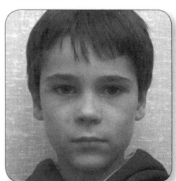

Control – Lips not rated

There are no limits or calculations to define full lips. Full lips, like many facial features are a visual impression. Assess the lips from a non-smiling photograph as smiling pulls the lips making them look thinner.

LIPS

Lips full - Red

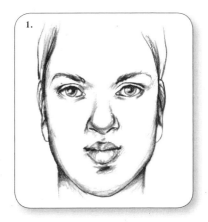
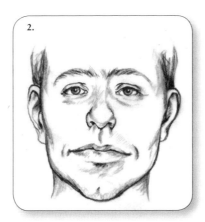
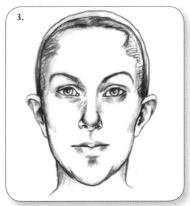
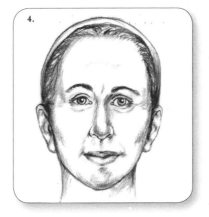

1. Lips full with a small mouth. This mouth will get two points. Full lips (red) and small mouth (yellow).

2. Lips full with a wide mouth. This mouth will get two points. Full lips (red) and wide mouth (red).

3. Top lip normal and bottom lip full giving overall impression of full lips (red).

4. Lips full with no other miasmatic rating to the mouth (red).

SMILE

Smile compact smile — Yellow

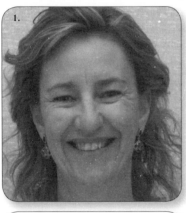

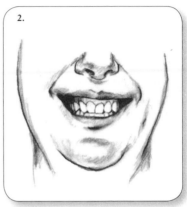

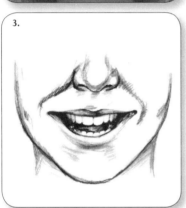

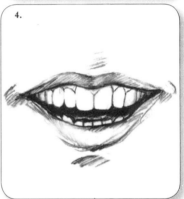

In a compact smile, the curve of the dental arch is narrow. When smiling, the lips and mouth stretch further than the teeth. Therefore, on smiling, the observer sees a space between the teeth and the inside of the mouth. This is because the dental arch is smaller and more 'compact'.

1. Compact smile with crossed over teeth. This smile will get two points Compact smile (yellow) and crossed over teeth (blue).
2. Compact smile with gums showing. This smile will get two points. Compact smile (yellow) and gums showing on smile (red).
3. Compact smile (yellow).
4. Smile not rated. The teeth in this example do not extend the full width of the mouth and there is not enough shadow to make them compact.

SMILE

Smile full — Red

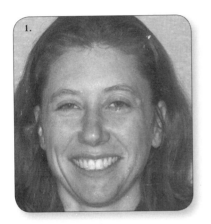
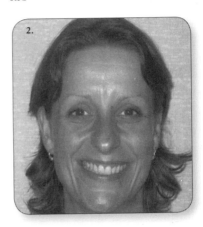

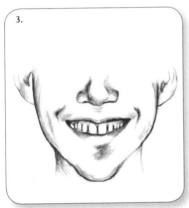
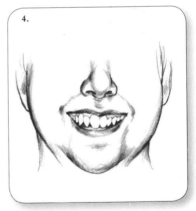

If the teeth fill the whole of the mouth while smiling it is termed a full smile. The mouth has no space that is not taken up by the teeth.

1. Full smile with even teeth. This mouth will get two points. Full smile (red) and even teeth (red).

2. Full smile with even teeth. This mouth will get two points. Full smile (red) and even teeth (red).

3. Full smile with gaps between the teeth. This mouth will get two points. Full smile (red) and gapped teeth (red).

4. Full smile with crooked teeth. This mouth will get two points. Full smile (red) and crooked teeth (blue).

SMILE

Smile large — Red

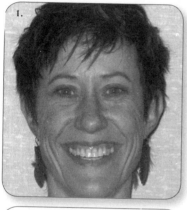
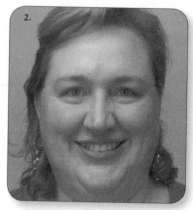
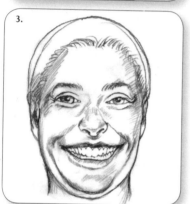
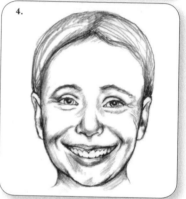

A smile that is eye catching and large when compared to other facial features is red. When the lips are closed, a person's mouth may be of average size yet when they smile it dominates the face.

.. Large smile (red).

!. Smile not rated.

i. Large smile (red). This smile extends almost the full width of the face.

. Large smile (red). This smile is large compared to other facial features.

SMILE

Smile gums — Red

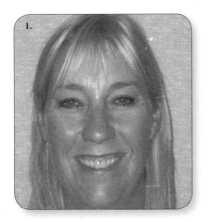

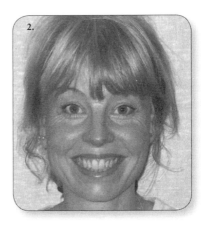

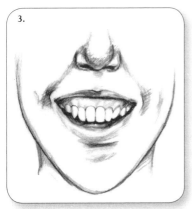

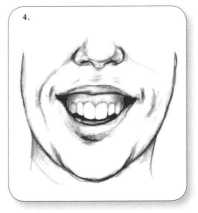

When a person smiles and the gums are obvious and prominent, one red point is given for that feature. Visible gums on smiling have nothing to do with the shape of the teeth.

1. Gums show on smiling (red).

2. Gums not rated.

3. Gums show on smiling with a full smile. This smile will get two points. Gums show on smiling (red) full smile (red).

4. Gums show on smiling with a compact smile. This smile will get two points. Gums show on smiling (red) compact smile (yellow).

TEETH

Teeth two front prominent — Yellow

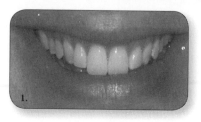

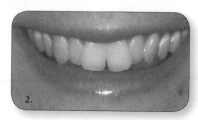

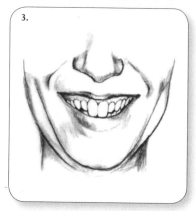

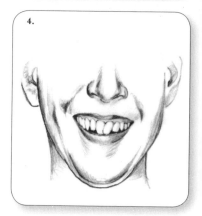

When the two front teeth look more prominent, large or forward than the teeth beside them (top row) they are yellow. This can give a 'rabbit' or 'bucky' appearance

1. The two front teeth are considerably longer than the other teeth (yellow).

2. The two front teeth stand out from the other teeth although not considerably longer (yellow).

3. Prominent front teeth longer (yellow).

4. Prominent front teeth larger with 'crossed-over' front teeth. These teeth will get two points. Prominent front teeth (yellow) and crossed over front teeth (blue).

TEETH

Teeth even — Red

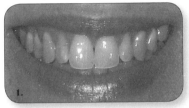

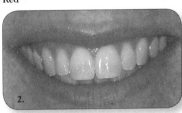

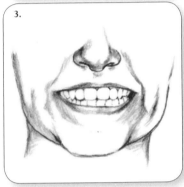

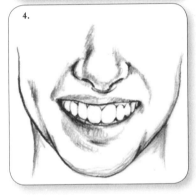

Firstly, check whether the patient has had dental braces and if so for what reason. Rate the teeth as they were BEFORE the dental work. Use old photos or the patient's memory. When analysing facial features we are analysing the physiological impact of the miasm they have inherited.

The typical even and often square teeth of red are what could be described as herbivorous teeth. They are large and even and sometimes spaced. They are designed for vegetable food unlike sharper teeth needed for meat.

1. Teeth even and full smile. These teeth will get two points. Teeth even (red) and full smile (red)

2. Teeth even and full smile. These teeth will get two points. Teeth even (red) and full smile (red)

3. Teeth even and square with a full smile. This smile will get two points. Teeth even (red) and full smile (red)

4. Teeth even but not square with a full smile. This smile will get two points. Teeth even (red) and full smile (red)

TEETH

Teeth gaps — Red

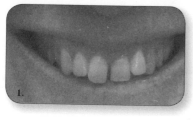

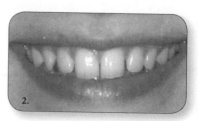

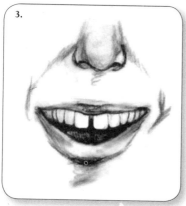

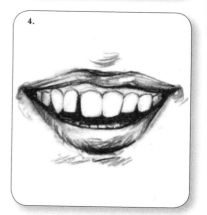

A single gap must be between the two front teeth in the top row. A single gap between any other teeth is not rated. Multiple gaps between the teeth are also given one red point.

1. Gap between the two front teeth (red)

2. Gaps between all teeth (red)

3. Gap between the two front teeth, even teeth and full smile. These teeth will get three points. Teeth gapped (red), teeth even (red) and smile full (red)

4. Single gap beside the front two teeth (not rated). This image is not rated for the smile or the shape or presentation of the teeth

TEETH

Teeth crooked — Blue

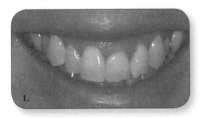

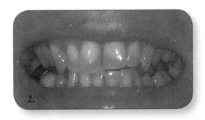

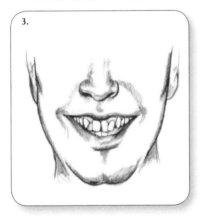

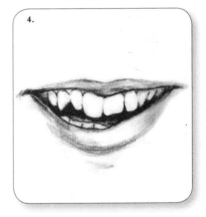

Crooked can mean uneven or it can mean asymmetrical. If crooked, the teeth are not equal in size nor do they sit in a straight line. If asymmetrical, the teeth are not the same shape. Both examples get one blue point.

1. Teeth that are different in size (blue).

2. Teeth that are crooked (blue).

3. Teeth that are crooked in both size, shape and direction (one blue point).

4. Teeth that are uneven and crooked (one blue point).

TEETH

Teeth sharp pointed — Blue

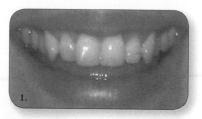

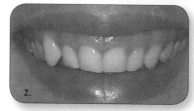

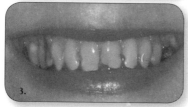

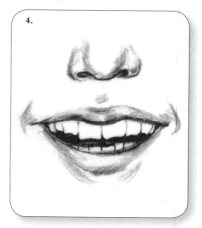

With sharp teeth, the teeth come to a point at their end rather than a normal flat edge. One sharp tooth in a mouthful of even teeth is not distinguishing enough to rate a blue point. At least both eyeteeth must be sharp to rate. Cupped teeth are rare but also get one blue point. In this feature, the edge of the teeth have a semi-circular inward arc rather than a straight edge.

1. Sharp eyeteeth with a full smile. These teeth will get two points. Sharp eyeteeth (blue) and full smile (red)

2. Sharp eyeteeth with gums on smiling. These teeth will get two points. Sharp eyeteeth (blue) and gums showing on smile (red)

3. Sharp, crooked teeth (one blue point)

4. Cupped teeth (blue)

TEETH

Teeth overbite — Blue

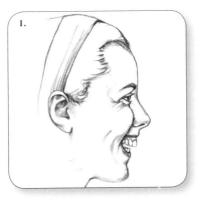

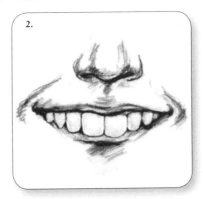

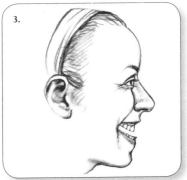

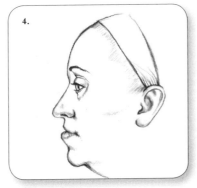

In an overbite, the top teeth extend beyond the lower teeth and create a space. Normally the top teeth fit tightly over the lower teeth, but an overbite extends beyond this to the point where the tip of the little finger will fit in the gap. In an under-bite the bottom teeth extend over the top teeth when the mouth is closed. An under-lip is also a blue feature although it occurs independently of the teeth. In an under-lip the bottom lip extends further out than the top lip where both should be even.

1. Overbite on profile (blue).

2. Overbite seen front on (blue).

3. Under-bite on profile (blue).

4. Under-lip on profile (blue).

TEETH

Teeth inward — Blue

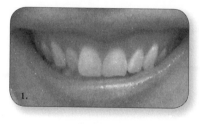 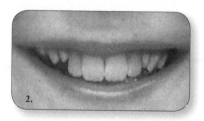

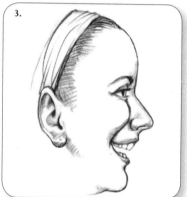 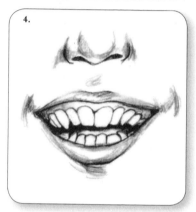

Teeth that angle into the mouth are inward teeth. Generally the front teeth are straight while the side teeth are inward, but sometimes all the teeth can be inward including the front although this is rare.

1. The front two teeth are straight but the remainder are angled inwards (blue)

2. The front four teeth are straight but the remainder are angled inwards (blue)

3. Inward teeth on profile (blue)

4. Inward teeth front on (blue)

TEETH

Teeth crossed — Blue

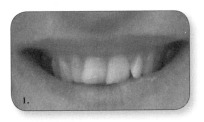

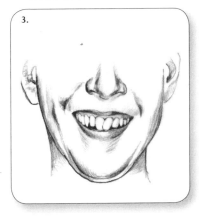

At the point of writing Appearance and Circumstance, the crossed over front teeth had only been seen in green patients. Therefore, it had to be either a blue or a yellow feature. Because of its affinity for the two front teeth, yellow seemed the most likely influence however over time, this has proved not to be the case and crossed front teeth indicates blue. Crossed over teeth usually occurs with the two front teeth but can occur with other teeth too.

1. Crossed front teeth with a yellow compact smile. This mouth will get two points. Crossed front teeth (blue) and compact smile (yellow).

2. Crossed front teeth with a full smile. These teeth will get two points. Crossed front teeth (blue) and full smile (red).

CHIN

Chin sloping - Yellow

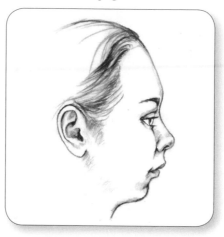

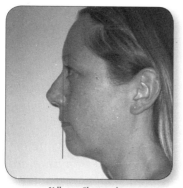

Yellow – Sloping chin

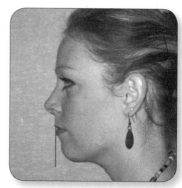

Yellow – Sloping chin

A sloping chin is seen on profile. The chin lies back from the mouth and often back from the bridge of the nose. From between the eyes, draw a hypothetical line vertically down the profile. This line highlights that the chin slopes back. A second point of reference to measure a sloping chin is a hypothetical line from the upper lip. The lower lip and chin should line up level to this vertical line. The sloping chin sits back from this point. However, for the vast majority of people, between the eyes is the best reference point to start with.

CHIN

Chin sloping - Yellow

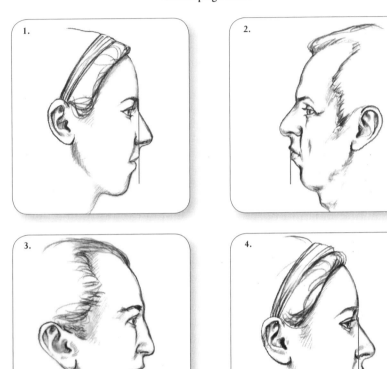

1. Line from between the eyes highlighting the sloping chin (yellow).

2. Line from upper lip highlighting the sloping chin (yellow).

3. Sloping chin without any defined bone structure. This is colloquially called 'chinless' (yellow).

4. Control with line from between the eyes – chin not rated.

CHIN

Chin ball - Red

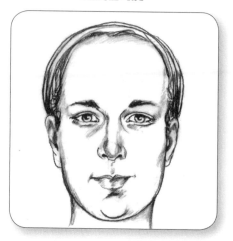

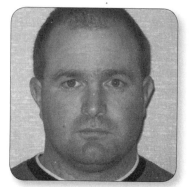
Red – Ball chin protruding

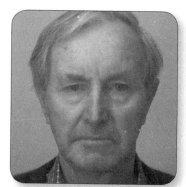
Red – Ball chin not protruding

The ball chin can take a number of forms. Most commonly, it is a circular protrusion from the chin but it may also be a circular shape or pattern without any protrusion. The circular shape lies flat against the surface of the skin, it is not raised and yet clearly visible.

CHIN

Chin ball - Red

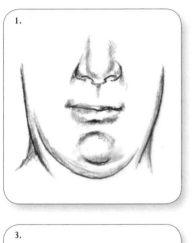

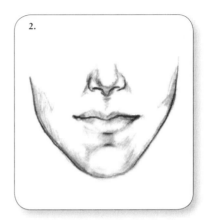

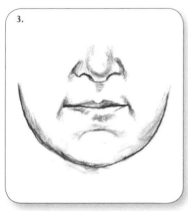

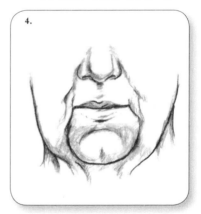

1. Ball chin protruding – with a raised surface area (red.)

2. Ball chin not protruding – without a raised surface area (red).

3. Ball chin defined by a single arched line below the mouth (red).

4. Ball chin with a cleft and defined. This chin will get three points. Ball (red) cleft (red) and defined (blue)

CHIN

Chin cleft - Red

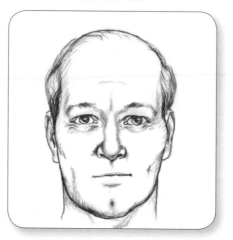

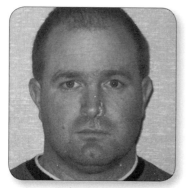

Red – Cleft in chin

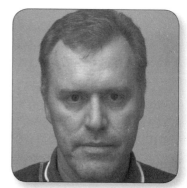

Control – Chin not rated

A cleft is a line or a dimple, located in the middle of the chin. Cleft has been used to avoid any confusion with blue dimples. Similar to lines, a cleft needs to be strong enough to be easily observable. Usually a cleft is seen in the middle fleshy part of the chin but sometimes will show in the bony edge of the chin.

CHIN

Chin cleft - Red

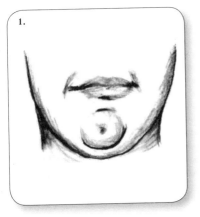

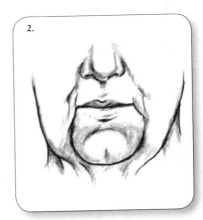

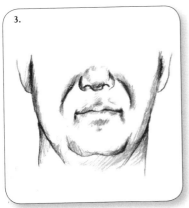

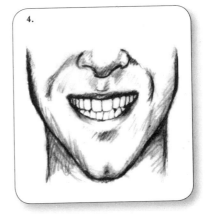

1. A cleft and a ball chin. This chin will get two points. Cleft (red) and ball chin (red).

2. A cleft, ball and a defined chin. This chin will get three points. Cleft (red) ball chin (red) and defined chin (blue).

3. A cleft in the bony edge of the chin (red).

4. A cleft and a pointed chin. This chin will get two points. Cleft (red) and pointed chin (blue).

CHIN

Chin defined/pointed - Blue

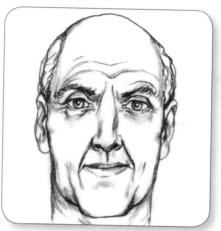

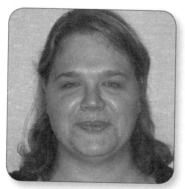

Blue – Chin defined

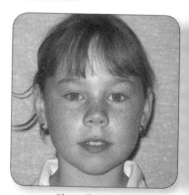

Blue – Chin pointed

A defined chin is where the bone structure of the chin looks separate from the jaw line creating a wide 'U' shape under the mouth. This shape can also be squared.

When the shape of the jaw forms a sharp tip at the chin, it is termed a pointed chin. Both a defined chin and a pointed chin are blue.

CHIN

Chin defined/pointed - Blue

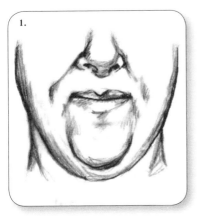

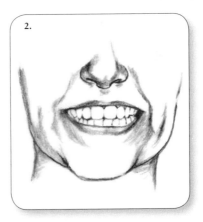

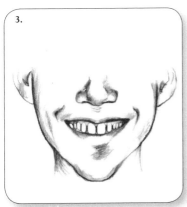

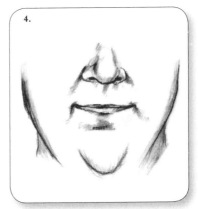

1.   Defined chin creating a 'U' shape under the mouth (blue).

2.   Defined chin creating a squared shape (blue).

3.   Pointed chin (blue).

4.   Pointed chin (blue).

EARS

Ears high – Yellow

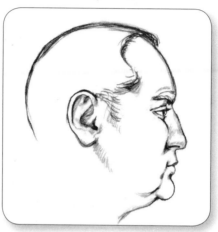

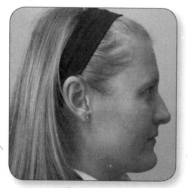

Yellow – Ears high

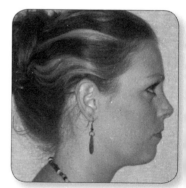

Control – Height not rated

Draw a hypothetical line on profile, from the bridge of the nose horizontally towards the back of the head. This line should be equal with the upper eyelids as well as the top of the ear. When the top of the ear is visibly higher than this mark, it rates one yellow point. Remember, that both ears need to be higher than this point otherwise, they are not rated. It is very important that the patient is holding their head straight or the ear position can look different to what it really is. Ears can look high or low from a front on position but must only be measured on profile.

EARS

Ears high – Yellow

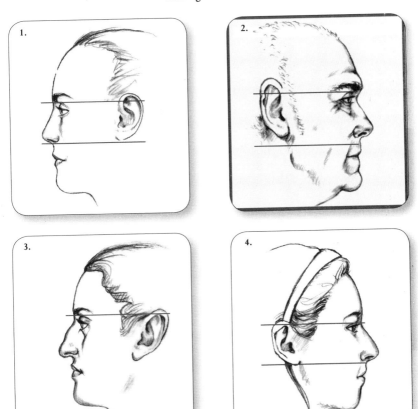

1. High ears showing reference point (yellow)
2. High ears which are also large. These ears will get two points.
    High ears (yellow) and large ears (blue)
3. High ears sloping back. These ears will get two points. High
    (yellow) and sloped back (yellow)
4. Ears on the borderline of average height (not rated)

EARS

Ears low – Yellow

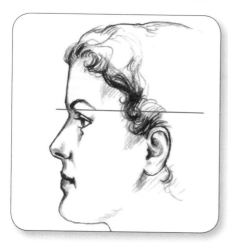

When the top of the ear is visibly lower than this line, it rates one yellow point.

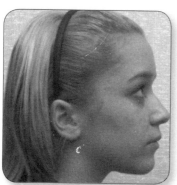

Yellow – Ears low

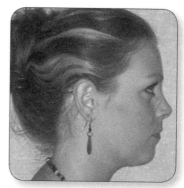

Control – Height not rated

Sometimes ears can look low or high from a front on position but ears can only be measured properly on profile only. Remember, that both ears need to be lower than this point otherwise, they are asymmetrical and not yellow. It is very important that the patient is holding their head straight or the ear position can look different to what it really is. Ears can look high or low from a front on position but must only be measured on profile.

EARS

Ears low – Yellow

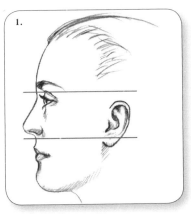

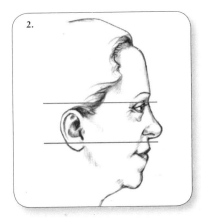

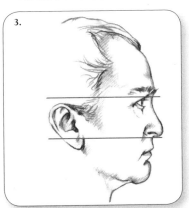

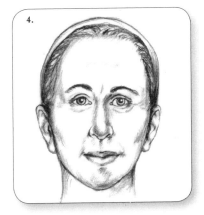

1. Low ears showing reference point (yellow)

2. Low ears which are also small. These ears will rate two points. Low ears (yellow) and small ears blue)

3. Low ears sloping back. These ears will get two points. Low (yellow) and sloped back (yellow)

4. Low ears seen front on (yellow)

EARS

Ears sloped – Yellow

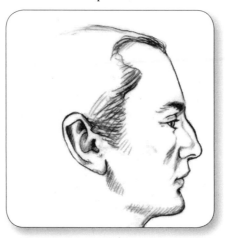

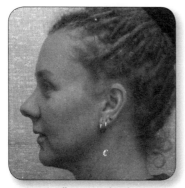

Yellow – Ears sloped

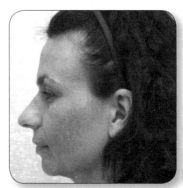

Control – Slope not rated

Drawing a line from the inner edge of the lower lobe of the ear upward, the edge of the upper part of the ear should rest just behind this line. When it is twenty degrees or more behind this line, the ears are sloped.

EARS

Ears sloped – Yellow

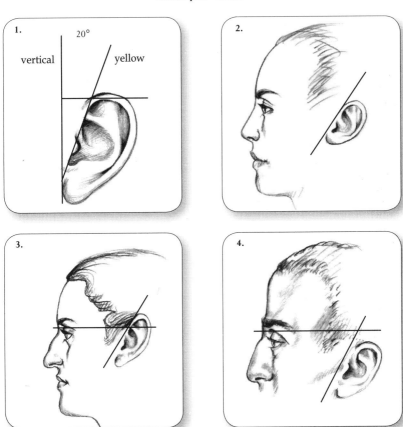

1. Sloping ears (yellow) – showing reference point.
2. Sloping ear (yellow).
3. Sloping ears that are also high. These ears will get two points. Sloped (yellow) and high (yellow).
4. Sloping ears that are also low. These ears will get two points. Sloped (yellow) and low (yellow).

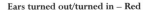

EARS

Ears turned out/turned in – Red

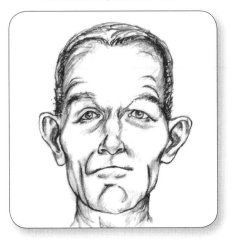

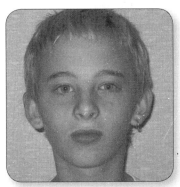
Red – Ears turned out

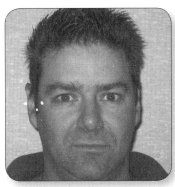
Control – Ears not rated

Turned out ears are those that extend outward from the head. Rather than flat to the side of the head, the ears project outward and face toward the front.

Ears turned in describes ears that are outward (when observed front on) for half of their length then curve in towards the head.

EARS

Ears turned out/turned in – Red

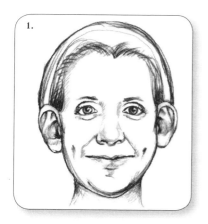

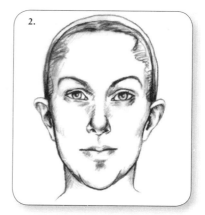

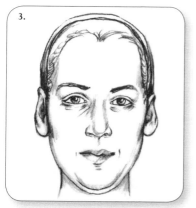

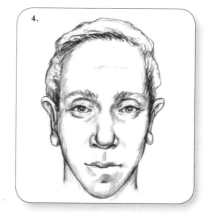

1. Ears turned out along the whole ear (red).
2. Ears turned out at the top (red).
3. Ears turned in (red).
4. Ears turned out both top and bottom (red).

EARS

Ears large – Blue

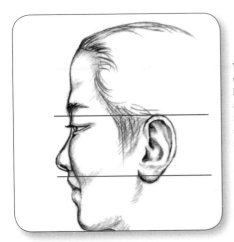

When the top of the ear is above the upper line and/or below the lower line it is usually large. Sometimes an ear is still large even if it doesn't fit outside these lines – this is a visual image by comparison to average sized ears.

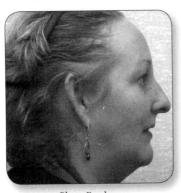

Blue – Ears large

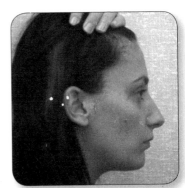

Control – Ears not rated for size

An ear can be high or low and/or large or small. Look at both height and size. The two measurements are separate and don't always go with one another. The size of ears is best measured on profile. If the lobes are very stretched from heavy earrings estimate the ear size as if they were not stretched.

EARS

Ears large – Blue

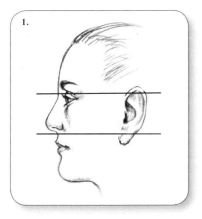

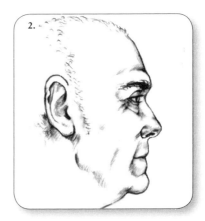

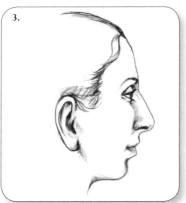

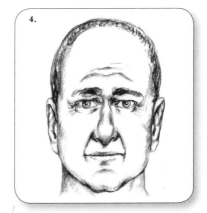

1. Lines showing reference point for large ears (blue)

2. Large ears that are high. These ears will get two points. Large (blue) and high (yellow)

3. Large ears that are low. These ears will get two points. Large (blue) and low (yellow)

4. Large ears front on (blue)

EARS ·

Ears small – Blue

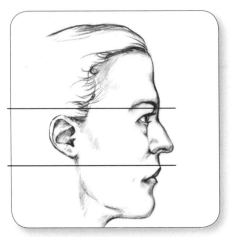

When the top of the ear is below the upper line and/or above the lower line it is usually small. Sometimes an ear is still small even if it doesn't fit within these lines – this is a visual image by comparison to average sized ears.

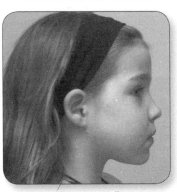

Blue – Ears Small

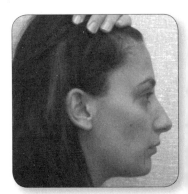

Control – Ears not rated for size

An ear can be high or low and/or large or small. Look at both height and size. The two measurements are separate and don't always go with one another. The size of ears is best measured on profile. If the lobes are very stretched from heavy earrings estimate the ear size as if they were not stretched.

EARS

Ears small – Blue

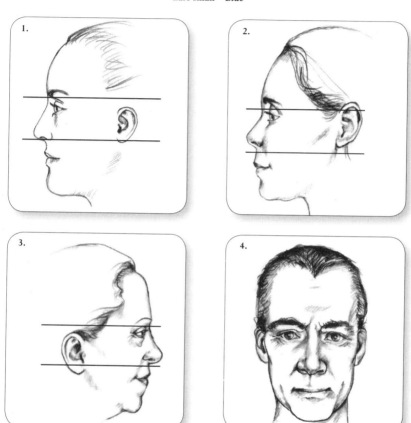

1. Lines showing reference point for small ears (blue).

2. Small ears that are high. These ears will get two points. Small (blue) and high (yellow).

3. Small ears that are low. These ears will get two points. Small (blue) and low (yellow).

4. Small ears shown front on (blue).

LINES

Lines forehead – Yellow

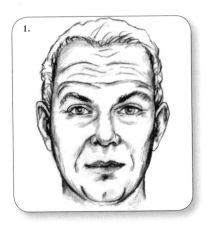

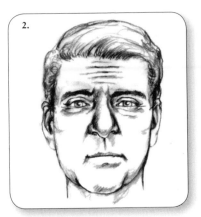

These are lines commonly termed worry lines. They are positioned either across the forehead or in the middle just above the eyes. Most people when they frown or look surprised have lines in their forehead, so the determining factor is how deeply etched they are. If they are faint they are not worthy of consideration and should be left out. However, if they are strong and eye catching, they should be included as one yellow point. Commonly these lines take the shape of a wave rather than straight but either count as one yellow point.

1.   Multiple lines across forehead in a wave shape (yellow)

2.   Multiple lines in the middle of the forehead (yellow)

LINES

Lines below the eyes – Yellow

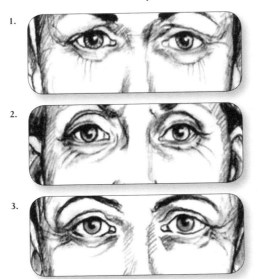

Most adults will have lines at the corner of their eyes especially when they smile, these are colloquially referred to as 'crows feet'. Separate to these are the lines that lie under the eyes. These lines extend downwards from the lower lid of the eye, from the outer canthus inward to approximately one third of the width of the eye. These lines extend directly downward or slant slightly at an angle away from the eye.

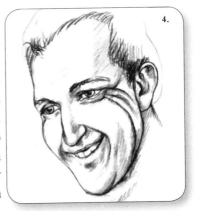

If very deep, these lines may extend to the cheeks, this generally occurs only when smiling.

1. Lines extending directly downward from the eyes (yellow).

2. Lines below eyes (yellow).

3. Normal crows feet (not rated).

4. Lines extending to cheeks (yellow).

LINES

Lines between eyes two — Yellow

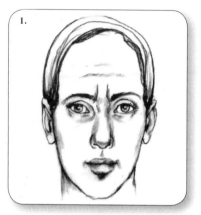

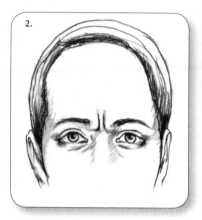

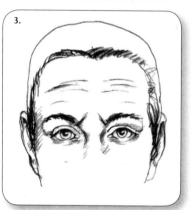

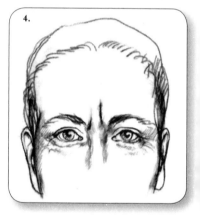

Two lines between the eyes indicate yellow. Like all lines, they are judged by their depth and are often seen during the consultation when the patient is animated rather than by photo.

1. Two lines extending from the eyebrows (yellow).

2. Two lines from between the eyebrows (yellow).

3. Two lines diagonally inward (yellow).

4. Two lines unequal length but both prominent (yellow).

Footnote - 3 lines between eyes is also a yellow feature (no sketch)

LINES

Lines between eyes one — Red

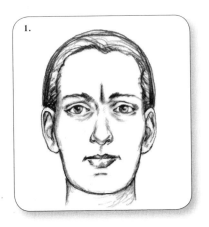
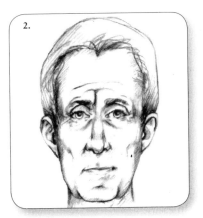

The single line is one etched line that commences between the eyebrows. Generally this single line is straight and centred but can also be seen slightly left or right of centre. Like all lines, they are judged by their depth and are often seen during the consultation when the patient is animated rather than by photo.

1. Single line centred (red)
2. Single line off centre (red)

LINES

Lines around mouth — Red

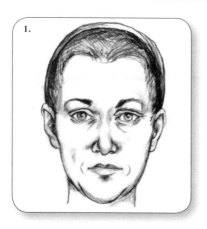

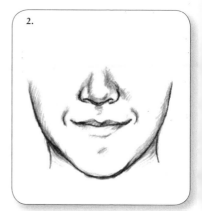

These lines are usually about one centi-metre long and have a crescent moon shape. They sit just outside the corners of the mouth. On smiling they will be deeper but their size and shape remain the same.

1. Lines around the mouth, a common example (red).
2. Lines around the mouth on smiling (red).

LINES

Line across bridge — Blue

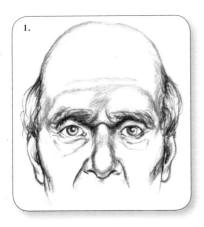 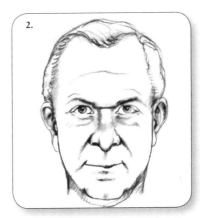

This line is either straight and horizontal or a semi-circular curve that stretches from one side of the bridge of the nose to the other. This line is often associated with an indented bridge. This line is counted even if it isn't deep.

1. Horizontal line that is curved (blue).

2. Horizontal line that is straight (blue).

LINES

Lines/dimples in cheeks — Blue

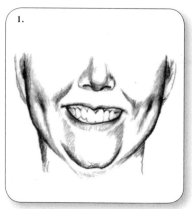

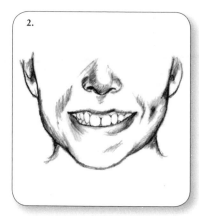

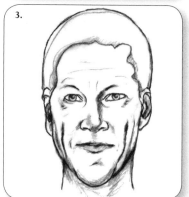

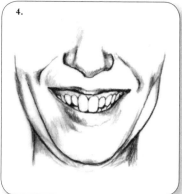

Dimples are usually only seen when a person smiles, however sometimes they can be so deep that their outline is seen when not smiling. One dimple or two dimples - both are rated as one blue point.

Separate to dimples are strong long lines in the cheeks. If a person is overweight, be careful not to take the line of the jaw as a line in their cheeks. The extra fat of the double chin will create this illusion.

1. Dimples seen on smiling (blue)

2. Single dimple (blue)

3. Lines in the cheeks (blue)

4. Dimples merging into a line (one blue point)

LINES

Lines down from nose — Blue

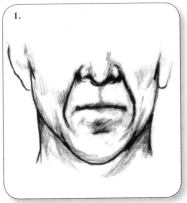

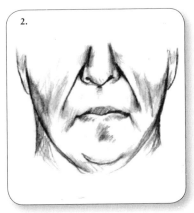

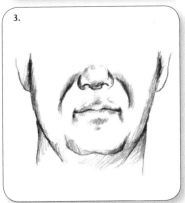

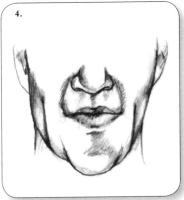

Beginning from the corners of the nose these lines extend downward to just outside the corners of the mouth or slightly below. These lines may be straight but most commonly are curved. Occasionally these lines do not extend to the corners of the mouth but finish at the upper lip.

1. Lines extending from the corners of the nose to below the corners of the mouth (blue)

2. Lines straight from corners of nose (blue)

3. Lines curved downward but not reaching the mouth (blue)

4. Lines curved downward from beside the nose reaching the mouth (blue)

LINES

Line down from the mouth — Blue

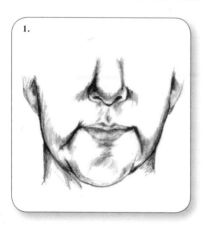

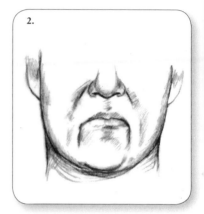

These lines begin at the corners of the mouth and extend downward at a slight angle toward the jaw.

1. Lines down from the mouth slightly angled (blue).

2. Lines straight down from the mouth (blue).

SKIN

Skin freckles/lines — Yellow

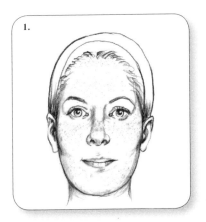 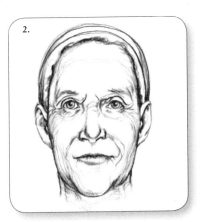

Freckles are a yellow skin feature however; the freckles must be numerous and cover most of the surface area of the face. One or a few freckles including a sprinkling of freckles across the nose is not enough to register, they must cover the whole face and be easily noticeable.

Multiple fine lines in the skin, either all over the face or in the cheeks are yellow.

1.   An example of freckles (yellow)

2.   An example of multiple fine lines in the face especially the cheeks (yellow)

ASYMMETRY

Asymmetry – Blue

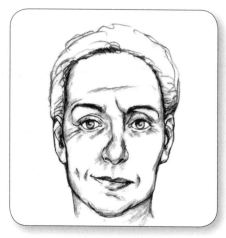

Asymmetry is when one facial feature has a different shape, size or position than its counterpart. An eye that is higher, a nose that bends, or a smile that pulls to one side.

Asymmetry is allocated from <u>four features only</u> — eyes, nose, mouth and chin. It can be subtle but it is important that it is not too subtle.

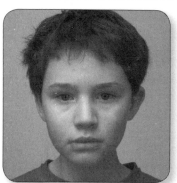

Blue – Asymmetry one point

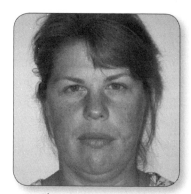

Blue – Asymmetry two points

Asymmetry is rated according to its frequency. Asymmetry exists in every person's face, so one asymmetrical feature is not strong enough to rate. Two or three asymmetrical features rate one blue point, while four or more asymmetrical features rates two blue points.

Photo 1 — Asymmetry in mouth and height of eyes — one blue point.
Photo 2 — Asymmetry in height of eyes, curve of nose, mouth pulled to her right and chin pulled to her left – two blue points.

ASYMMETRY

Asymmetry – Blue

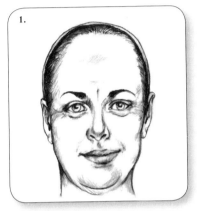

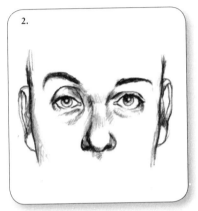

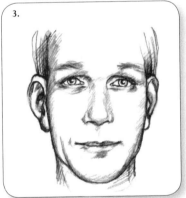

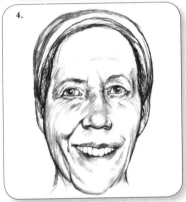

All sides are from the perspective of the patient.

1. Asymmetry – left eye higher, mouth pulled to left = 1 point (blue).

2. Asymmetry – eyes – position and lids (blue)*.

3. Asymmetry – eyes and nose (blue).

4. Asymmetry – the eyes are a different size, the nose is curved, the mouth is pulled to the right and the chin pulls to the right = 2 points (blue).

*occasionally one feature has two aspects that are asymmetrical= 1 point (blue)

YELLOW

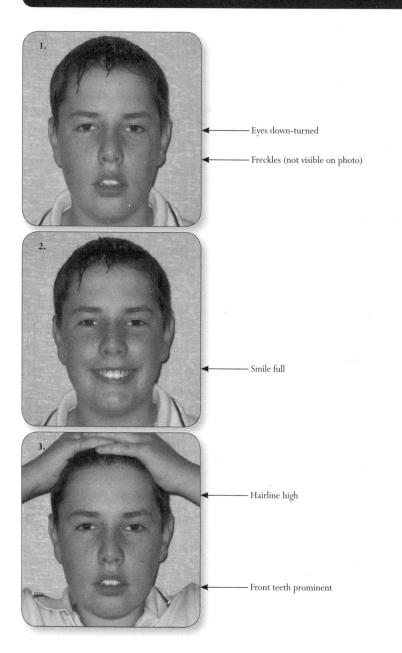

1. — Eyes down-turned

— Freckles (not visible on photo)

2. — Smile full

3. — Hairline high

— Front teeth prominent

YELLOW

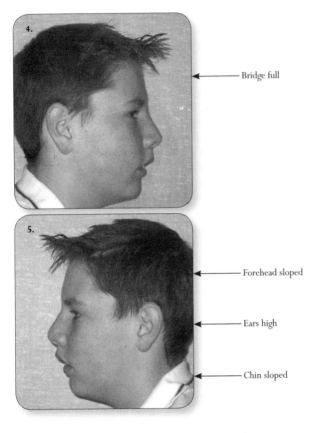

4.
— Bridge full

5.
— Forehead sloped

— Ears high

— Chin sloped

YELLOW - 6	RED - 2	BLUE - 1
Eyes down-turned	Smile full	Hairline high
Freckles	Bridge full	
Front teeth prominent		
Forehead sloped		
Ears high		
Chin sloped		

ORANGE

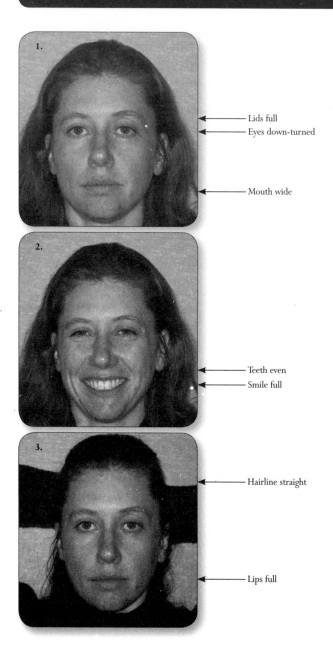

1.
— Lids full
— Eyes down-turned

— Mouth wide

2.
— Teeth even
— Smile full

3.
— Hairline straight

— Lips full

ORANGE

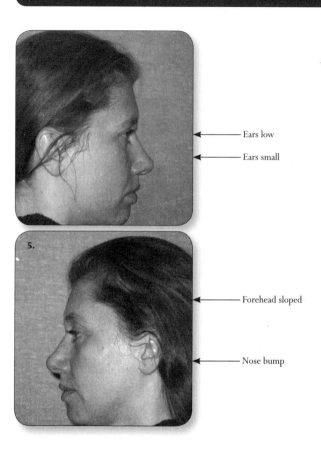

Ears low
Ears small

Forehead sloped

Nose bump

YELLOW - 5	RED - 5	BLUE - 1
Forehead sloped	Hairline straight	Ears small
Lids full	Mouth wide	
Eyes down-turned	Smile full	
Ears low	Teeth even	
Nose bump	Lips full	

RED

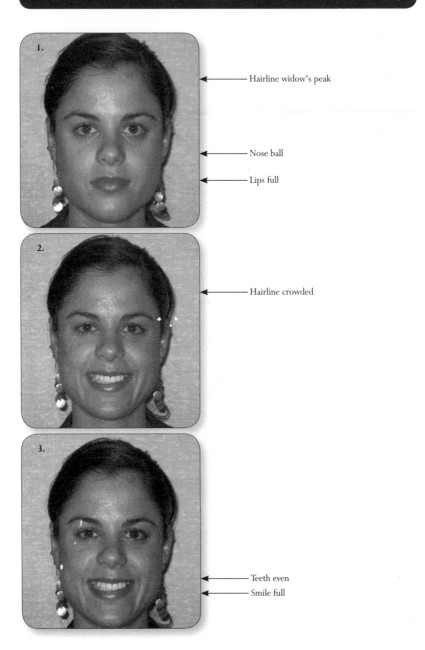

1.
— Hairline widow's peak

— Nose ball

— Lips full

2.
— Hairline crowded

3.
— Teeth even
— Smile full

RED

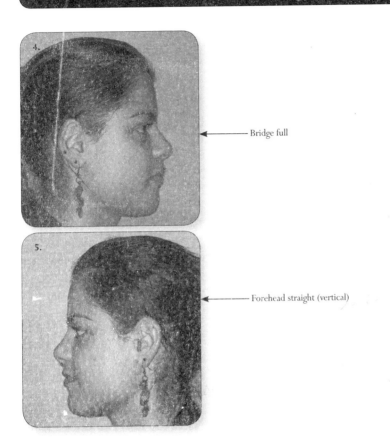

Bridge full

Forehead straight (vertical)

YELLOW - 1	RED - 7	BLUE - 0
Hairline widow's peak	Hairline crowded	
	Forehead straight (vertical)	
	Bridge full	
	Nose ball	
	Lips full	
	Teeth even	
	Smile full	

PURPLE

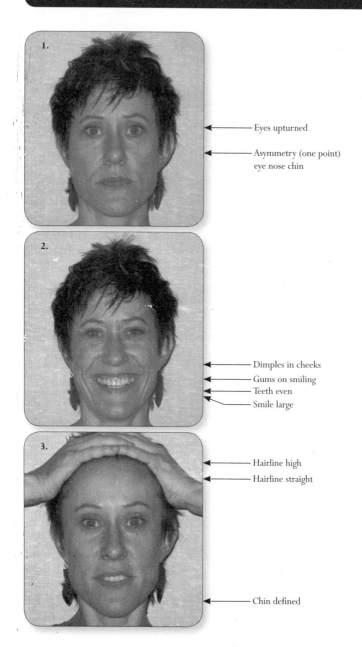

1.

Eyes upturned

Asymmetry (one point)
eye nose chin

2.

Dimples in cheeks
Gums on smiling
Teeth even
Smile large

3.

Hairline high
Hairline straight

Chin defined

PURPLE

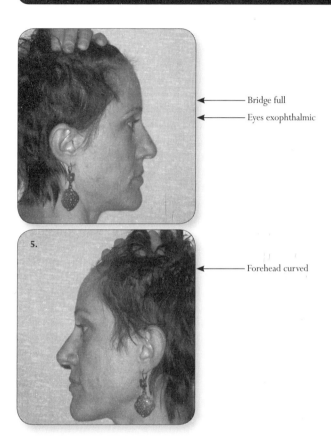

Bridge full
Eyes exophthalmic

Forehead curved

YELLOW - 0	RED - 6	BLUE - 6
	Hairline straight	Hairline high
	Bridge full	Forehead curved
	Eyes exophthalmic	Eyes upturned
	Gums on smiling	Asymmetry (eye,
	Teeth even	ncse, chin)
	Smile large	Dimples in cheeks
		Chin defined

BLUE

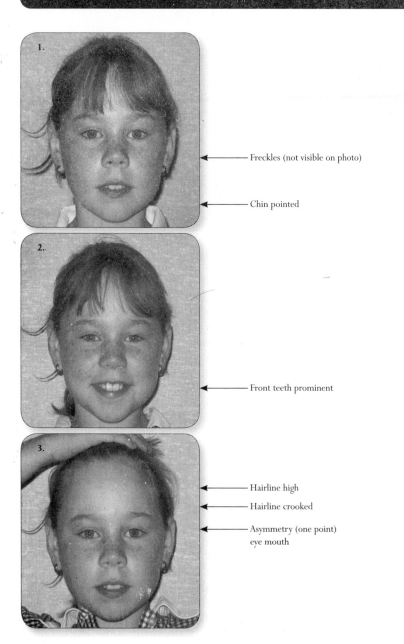

1.

Freckles (not visible on photo)

Chin pointed

2.

Front teeth prominent

3.

Hairline high

Hairline crooked

Asymmetry (one point)
eye mouth

BLUE

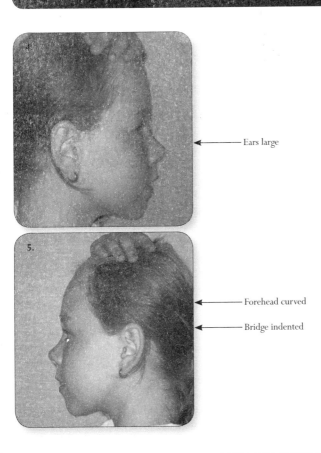

Ears large

Forehead curved

Bridge indented

YELLOW - 2	RED - 0	BLUE - 7
Freckles Front teeth prominent		Hairline high Hairline crooked Forehead curved Bridge indented Asymmetry (eyes, mouth) Chin pointed Ears large

GREEN

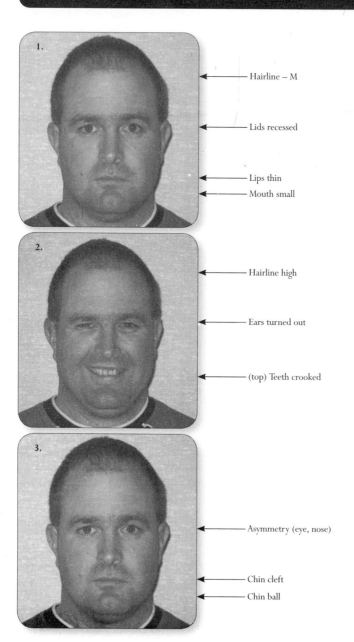

1.
- Hairline – M
- Lids recessed
- Lips thin
- Mouth small

2.
- Hairline high
- Ears turned out
- (top) Teeth crooked

3.
- Asymmetry (eye, nose)
- Chin cleft
- Chin ball

GREEN

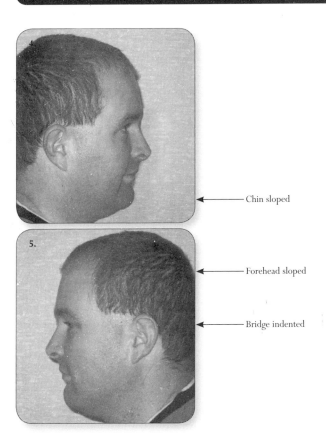

Chin sloped

5.

Forehead sloped

Bridge indented

YELLOW - 5	RED - 3	BLUE - 5
Hairline – M	Chin cleft	Hairline high
Forehead sloped	Chin ball	Lids recessed
Mouth small	Ears turned out (top)	Asymmetry (eye, ear, nose)
Lips thin		Teeth crooked
Chin sloped		Bridge indented

BROWN

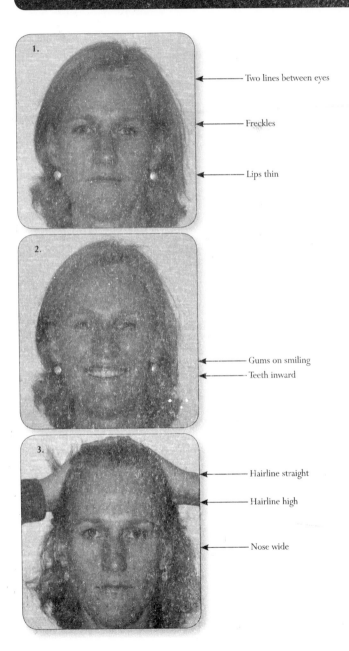

1. Two lines between eyes
   Freckles
   Lips thin

2. Gums on smiling
   Teeth inward

3. Hairline straight
   Hairline high
   Nose wide

BROWN

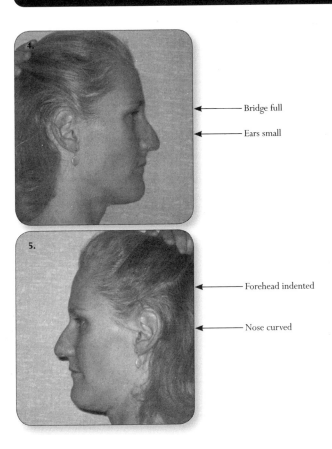

4.
— Bridge full
— Ears small

5.
— Forehead indented
— Nose curved

YELLOW - 4	RED - 4	BLUE - 4
Two lines between eyes	Hairline straight	Hairline high
Nose curved	Bridge full	Forehead indented
Freckles	Nose wide	Teeth inward
Lips thin	Gums on smiling	Ears small

CHART OF FEATURES

TYPE	YELLOW	RED	BLUE
Hairline	Widows peak M shape	Straight Low Crowded	High/Balding Crooked
Forehead	Sloped (straight 12º or greater)	Straight (vertical to 11º) Brow strong	Curved Indented
Bridge		Full/Straight	Indented
Eyes	Down-turned Close-set Small Full lids	Large Exophthalmic	Upturned Wide-set Deep-set Recessed lids Eye indents - new feature see HFA online course
Nose	Down-turned Curved Bump	Wide Ball Cleft+	
Cheeks			Bones strong Sunken under
Mouth	Small	Wide	
Lips	Thin	Full	Under-lip (profile)
Smile	Compact	Full Large Gums show	
Teeth	Front two prominent	Even Gaps (between front teeth or multiple)	Crooked Cross over front two* Sharp/pointed Cupped Overbite Under bite Inward
Chin	Sloped back	Ball Cleft	Defined Pointed

Ears	High Low Sloped	Turned out Turned in	Large Small
Lines	Forehead Eyes – below Eyes – two between Cheeks – multiple fine	Eyes – one between Mouth – around	Bridge – horizontal Cheeks – dimples/ lines Nose – down from Mouth – down from Eye indentations**
Asymmetry			Eyes, nose, mouth and chin 2 or 3 places = 1 point 4 places = 2 points
Skin	Freckles		

+ No example in book

* Classified incorrectly as yellow in Appearance and Circumstance– since confirmed as blue

** New feature 2009 – no picture in book–see HFA online course- www. vcch.org

FEATURES UPDATE 2006

When Appearance and Circumstance was published in 2003 we categorized 80 features. In this book we focus on slightly less features – for those who make a close comparison of the differences, the following are our findings. In some cases we have changed the terminology, in others we have dropped the feature due to its rarity or lack of definition.

CHANGE OF MIASM

Teeth – front two crossed over	The only feature mistakenly classified. Blue - not yellow

NEW NAMES

FEATURE	CURRENT STATUS
Hair – crowded in or squeezed at temples	Now known as crowded hairline – where the hair crowds in at the side of the hairline near the temples – not literally squeezed in temples. Often seen with a low hairline although not always.

FEATURES NO LONGER USED

FEATURE	CURRENT STATUS
Eyes – focus off centre*	Difficult to define so we have dropped this feature.
Eyes – round	Difficult to define so we have dropped this feature.
Eyes – almond	Difficult to define so we have dropped this feature.
Nose – ski-jump	Difficult to define so we have dropped this feature. Nose ball shape - one red point – seen front on or on profile – same shape
Nose – snubbed	Rarely seen we have dropped this feature.

Nose – saddle	Difficult to define so we have dropped this feature. It was originally intended as an indented shape in the bone structure – rarely seen and often misunderstood as a skin pattern. We have dropped this feature.
Teeth – square	Almost always seen in conjunction with even teeth so one red feature is given for even. The square shape has been dropped to avoid doubling up.
Face – flat	Too difficult to define so we have dropped this feature – it is easier to analyse each part separately.
Jaw – square	Too difficult to define so we have dropped this feature.
Skin – dry	Dryness is a sensation rather than a look – if the skin is yellow it will be seen in the lines. Persons of any miasm can have dry skin.
Skin – flushed	The colour of the skin varies due to racial background and state of health. We have dropped this feature.
Skin – excessive hair growth	Too difficult to determine due to cosmetic practices. This feature can also be related to the state of health. We have dropped this feature.
Skin – moles	Use this as confirmatory feature only (red) but not as part of the analysis.
Eyebrows	Too difficult to define so we have dropped this feature.
White of sclera	Too difficult to define so we have dropped this feature.

* Eyes - focus off centre was reintroduced in 2010 as a red feature - see HFA online course www.vcch.org

SAMUEL HAHNEMANN

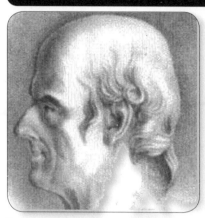

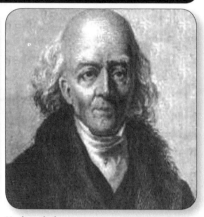

Forehead - curved
Nose - indented bridge
Nose- bump and down-turned
Cheeks -vertical lines

Hairline - high
Eyes - down-turned Eyes - deep-set
Mouth - small
Ears - low

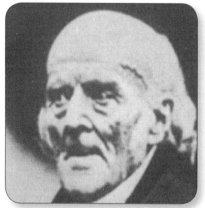

Only known photo taken in his late 80s [Photographs copyright Homeopathe Inte rnational]

YELLOW	RED	BLUE
Nose -long and curved		Forehead - curved
Lips- thin		Eyes - deep-set
Mouth - small		Lines - downturned from corners of mouth
Ears -sloping back/low		Cheeks - lines Hairline - high Cheekbones -prominent
Lines - 2 between eyes		nent
TOTAL		
5	0	6

Based on the above portraits and photograph, the most
likely deduction is that Samuel Hahnemann belonged to the

BIBLIOGRAPHY

Part 1 – Miasms

1 METHODOLOGY

Allen, J H, *The Chronic Miasms Vol. 1 – Psora and Pseudo-Psora*, Author, Chicago, 1910; reprint, B Jain Publishers, New Delhi, 1994.

Banerjea, Dr Subrata Kumar, *Miasmatic Diagnosis: Practical Tips with Clinical Comparisons*, B Jain Publishers, New Delhi, India, 1991.

Close, Stuart, *The Genius of Homoeopathy*, Homeopathic Publications, New Delhi,

Foubister, Donald, *The Carcinosin Drug Picture*, Macrepertory Reference Works

Hahnemann, Samuel, Wheeler, C E (trans.) *Organon of the Rational Art of Healing*, J M Dent & Sons, London, 1913.

Kent, J T, *Lectures on Homoeopathic Philosophy*, Thorsons Publishers Limited, Wellingborough, 1979.

Roberts, *The Principles and Art of Cure by Homoeopathy*, Health Science Press, Whitstable, Kent, 1942.

Stokes, John H, *Modern Clinical Syphilology: Diagnosis, Treatment, Case Studies*, W B Saunders, Philadelphia, 1926.

2 WHAT IS A MIASM?

Kent, J T, *New Remedies, Clinical Cases, Lesser Writings Aphorisms and Precepts*, Ehrhart & Karl, Chicago, 1926.

Kent, J T, *Lectures on Homoeopathic Philosophy*, Thorsons Publishers Limited, Wellingborough, 1979.

King, Serge Kahili, *Hawaiian Huna Shaman Training, Course Transcript* 'Tranceformations', 1990 (see also www.huna.org).

Ortega, Dr P S. *Notes on the Miasms* (1st English edn), National Homoeopathic Pharmacy, New Delhi, 1980.

Rinpoche, Sogyal, eds Patrick Gaffney and Andrew Harvey, *The*

Tibetan Book of Living and Dying, Rider, Random House, London, 1998.

3 HOMOEOPATHIC GENETICS – MIASMATIC INHERITANCE

Rinpoche, Sogyal, eds Patrick Gaffney and Andrew Harvey, *The Tibetan Book of Living and Dying*, Rider, Random House, London, 1998.

4 THE VARIOUS WAYS MIASM ARE CLINICALLY APPLIED

Hahnemann, Samuel, *Chronic Diseases: Their Peculiar Nature and Their Homoeopathic Cure*, B Jain Publishers, New Delhi, India, 1992.

Ortega, P S, *Notes on the Miasms*, National Homoeopathic Pharmacy, New Delhi, 1980.

Sankaran, Rajan, *Bombay Seminar 2002: Souvenir*, Homoeopathic Medical Publishers, Bombay, 2002

Vithoulkas, George, *The Science of Homoeopathy*, Vol. 1, ASOHM, Athens, 1978 (B Jain Publishers, reprint edn 1992).

5 THE SINGLE DOMINANT MIASM THEORY

Allen, J H, *The Chronic Miasms Vol. 1 – Psora and Pseudo-Psora*, Author, Chicago, 1910, 1994 reprint.

Boger, C M, *Collected Writings*, Churchill Livingstone, Edinburgh, 1994.

Hahnemann, Samuel, *Chronic Diseases: Their Peculiar Nature and Their Homoeopathic Cure*, B Jain Publishers, New Delhi, India, 1992.

6 PATHOLOGY AND THE MIASMS.

Close, S. *The Genius of Homoeopathy*, Homeopathic Publications, New Delhi.

Phatak, S R, *Materia Medica of Homoeopathic Medicines*, Indian Books and Periodicals Synd., New Delhi,1977.

7 THE NUMBER OF MIASMS

Allen, J H, *The Chronic Miasms Vol. 1 – Psora and Pseudo-Psora*, Author, Chicago, 1910, B Jain Publishers, 1994 reprint.

Boger, C M, *Collected Writings*, Churchill Livingstone, Edinburgh, 1994.

Campbell, A, *The Two Faces of Homoeopathy*, Robert Hale, London, 1984.

Hahnemann, Samuel, *Chronic Diseases: Their Peculiar Nature and Their Homoeopathic Cure*, B Jain Publishers, New Delhi, India, 1992.

Hahnemann, Samuel, Wheeler, C E (trans.) *Organon of the Rational Art of Healing*, J M Dent & Sons, London, 1913; 5th and 6th edition with Dudgeon, B Jain Publishers, 1992 (reprint edn).

MacRepertory 5.7, Complete 45 repertorization, skin-warts (see also www. repertory.org)

Morningstar, Sally, *Divining the Future: Discover and Shape Your Destiny by Interpreting Signs, Symbols and Dreams*, Anness Publishing Inc., 1998. Morrison, R, *Desktop Guide to Keynotes and Confirmatory Symptoms*

Hahnemann Clinic Publishing, Albany, 1993.

8 THE DEVELOPMENT OF THE NEW MIASMS

Handley, R, *In Search of the Later Hahnemann*, Beaconsdd Publishers Ltd, Beaconse l d, 1997.

Morrison, R, *Desktop Guide to Keynotes and Confirmatory Symptoms* Hahnemann Clinic Publishing, Albany, 1993.

Vermeulen, F, *Synoptic Materia Medica*, Merlijn Publishers, Haarlem, 1992.

9 FURTHER DEVELOPMENT OF THE EXISTING MIASMS

Handley, R, *In Search of the Later Hahnemann*, Beaconsdd Publishers Ltd, Beaconse l d, 1997.

Kent, J T, *Lectures on Homoeopathic Philosophy*, Thorsons Publishers Limited, Wellingborough, 1979.

10 COLOUR CODING THE MIASMS

Bleeding Gums Murphy, The Simpsons.

Hahnemann, Samuel, *Chronic Diseases: Their Peculiar Nature and Their Homoeopathic Cure*, B Jain Publishers, New Delhi, India, 1992. Kent, J T, *Lectures on Homoeopathic Philosophy*, Thorsons Publishers Limited, Wellingborough, 1979.

11 FACIAL FEATURES AS INDICATORS OF THE MIASM
Allen, J H, *The Chronic Miasms Vol. 1 – Psora and Pseudo-Psora*, Author, Chicago, 1910; reprint, B Jain Publishers, New Delhi, 1994.

12 HOW TO USE THE MIASMS IN CLINICAL PRACTICE
Woman the carrier of creation. Pub. McDonald Bayne Consultants. 1991 ed.

Kent, J T, *New Remedies, Clinical Cases, Lesser Writings Aphorisms and Precepts*, Ehrhart & Karl, Chicago, 1926.

Part 2 – Miasmatic Themes

14 MIASMATIC THEMES – PSORA (YELLOW)
Kent, J T, *Lectures on Homoeopathic Philosophy*, Thorsons Publishers Limited, Wellingborough, 1979.
MacRepertory 5.7, Complete 45 repertorization (see also www.repertory.org)

15 MIASMATIC THEMES – SYCOSIS (RED)
Banerjea, Dr Subrata Kumar, *Miasmatic Diagnosis: Practical Tips with Clinical Comparisons*, B Jain Publishers, New Delhi, India, 1991.
Luscher, Dr Max, and Scott, Ian A (ed), *The Luscher Color Test*, Jonathan Cape, 1970.
Vermeulen, F, *Synoptic Materia Medica*, Merlijn Publishers, Haarlem, 1992.

16 MIASMATIC THEMES – SYPHILIS (BLUE)
Luscher, Dr Max, and Scott, Ian A (ed), *The Luscher Color Test*, Jonathan Cape, 1970.

Nikiforuk, Andrew, *The Fourth Horseman*, Penguin Books, 1991 and 1996.

Roberts, *Principles and Art of Cure by Homoeopathy: A Modern Textbook* Homoeopathic Publishing Company, London, 1936.

17 MIASMATIC THEMES – SYCO-PSORA (ORANGE)

Luscher, Dr Max, and Scott, Ian A (ed), *The Luscher Color Test*, Jonathan Cape, 1970.

MacRepertory 5.7, Complete 45 repertorization (see also www.repertory.org)

Phatak, S R, *Materia Medica of Homoeopathic Medicines*, Indian Books and Periodicals Synd., New Delhi, 1977.]

18 MIASMATIC THEMES – SYCO-SYPHILIS (PURPLE)

Clarke, J H, *A Dictionary of Practical Materia Medica*, Homoeopathic Publishing Co., London, 1925. (New issue.). (ReferenceWorks).

Luscher, Dr Max, and Scott, Ian A (ed), *The Luscher Color Test*, Jonathan Cape, 1970.

MacRepertory 5.7, Complete 45 repertorization (see also www.repertory.org)

Zandvoort, Roger van, The Complete Repertory, Millenium Edition, ReferenceWorks.

19 MIASMATIC THEMES – TUBERCULAR (GREEN)

Luscher, Dr Max, and Scott, Ian A (ed), *The Luscher Color Test*, Jonathan Cape, 1970.

MacRepertory 5.7, Complete 45 repertorization (see also www.repertory.org)

Nikiforuk, Andrew, *The Fourth Horseman*, Penguine Books, 1991 and 1996.

Vermeulen, F, *Concordant Materia Medica*, Merlijn Publishers, Haarlem, 1994

20 MIASMATIC THEMES – CANCER (BROWN)

Clarke, J H, *A Dictionary of Practical Materia Medica*, Homoeopathic Publishing Co., London, 1925. (New issue.)

MacRepertory 5.7, Complete 45 repertorization (see also www.
    repertory.org)
Vermeulen, F, *Synoptic Materia Medica*, Merlijn Publishers, Haarlem,
    1992.

CONTACT US

We are happy to be contacted with your queries.

Contact us at admin@vcch.org

ADDRESS

Victorian College of Classical Homœopathy

PO Box 804

Mount Eliza Victoria Australia 3930

EMAIL : admin@vcch.org | **WEBSITE**: www.vcch.org

We will be updating the remedy list and adding any tips or new findings. There are some cases as examples of how facial analysis helps to choose remedies and more will be added as time permits

HOMEOPATHIC FACIAL ANALYSIS ONLINE COURSE

- Recorded online classes – 21 (at 2 hours each)
- Website notes – 400 pages
- Case examples – video and notes
- Available online for 18 months from date of enrolment

SPECIAL DISCOUNTED PRICE FOR INDIAN/SUBCONTINENT STUDENTS AND PRACTITIONERS

DISCOUNT ON REGULAR ENROLMENT FEE

http://www.vcch.org/india-special.html

FACIAL ANALYSIS SOFTWARE

A student/practitioner facial analysis software wizard is available

www.soulandsurvival.org/wizard/download

After a 10 day free trial the software must be purchased for continued use.

PRIVATE CONSULTATIONS (with Grant Bentley)

http://www.vcch.org/consultations.html